T0161498

THE ROAR BEHIND THE SILENCE
Why kindness, compassion and respect matter in maternity care

The Roar Behind the Silence:
Why kindness, compassion and respect matter in maternity care

First published by Pinter & Martin Ltd 2015
reprinted 2015

ISBN 978-1-78066-180-3
Also available as ebook

British Library Cataloguing-in-Publication Data
A catalogue record for this book is available from the British Library.

Set in Minion

Printed and bound in the UK by Martins the Printers, Berwick-upon-Tweed

Pinter & Martin Ltd
6 Effra Parade
London SW2 1PS

pinterandmartin.com

CONTENTS

I need *Catherine Grosvenor* 2

Foreword Hearing the roar behind the silence
Frances Day-Stirk, Sabaratnam Arulkumaran 7

Foreword *Toyin Saraki* 8

Introduction What's going on in maternity care?
Sheena Byrom, Soo Downe 9

Part I: Stories and perspectives from maternity care 13

1 Putting relationships at the heart of maternity care
   Penny Campling 15
2 Compassion in hospital care staff: what they think it is, what
   gets in its way, and how to enhance it *Michael Clift, Senga Steel* 21
3 Dignity in maternity: the power of human rights to improve
   care for childbearing women *Elizabeth Prochaska* 27
4 Only for the heartstrong *Olivia Armshaw* 31
5 When silence roars: Finley's stillbirth *Mel Scott* 38
6 Birth thoughts from Hungary: eternal gratitude *Anna Ternovszky* 44
7 Don't forget Dad! How does treating dads compassionately
   fit into woman-centred care? *Dean Beaumont* 48
8 Through the eyes of a doula *Kicki Hansard* 53
9 Promoting normal birth: courage through compassion
   Tracey Cooper 57
10 Not all obstetricians *Alison Barrett* 62
11 We can learn to be caring *Robin Youngson* 67

Part II: Principles and theories 77

12 Human rights principles in maternal health
   Diana Bowser, Mande Limbu 79
13 How kindness, warmth, empathy and support promote the
   progress of labour: a physiological perspective
   Kerstin Uvnäs Moberg 86
14 Spirituality, compassion and maternity care *Jenny Hall* 94
15 Stop the fear and embrace birth
   Hannah Dahlen, Kathryn Gutteridge 98
16 How environment and context can influence capacity
   for kindness *Mavis Kirkham* 105
17 Caring for ourselves: the key to resilience
   Billie Hunter, Lucie Warren 111

Part III: Making it happen: solutions from around the world   117

18 Clinical guidelines: hindrance or help for respectful compassionate care? *Julie Frohlich, Rineke Schram*   119

19 Making it happen in China *Ngai Fen Cheung*   127

20 Making it happen in Brazil *Maria Helena Bastos*   132

21 Making it happen in Catalonia, Spain *Ramón Escuriet*, Translation *Roberto Ortíz*   140

22 Italy, where is your beauty? *Laura Iannuzzi, Sandra Morano*   147

23 A good birth in the Netherlands *Raymond De Vries, Marijke Hendrix, Tamar van Haaren*   152

24 Open disclosure: a perspective from Ireland *Deirdre Munro*   157

25 They don't know what they don't know *Amali Lokugamage, Theresa Bourne*   162

26 With-woman, with-student: developing a woman and family-centred midwifery recruitment strategy and curriculum for caring *Anna Byrom, Shelagh Heneghan, Mercedes Perez-Bottella*   168

27 Care and compassion count: supporting student midwives in practice *Carmel McCalmont, Sue Lees*   177

28 Compassionate care, midwives, women and forum theatre: two tales from practice *Adele Stanley, Gemma Boyd, Anna Byrom, Kirsten Baker*   181

29 Moving to positive childbirth *Milli Hill*   189

30 Walking in another's shoes *Gill Phillips*   196

31 Compassion in the social era *Teresa Chinn*   201

32 Kindness is a cost-effective solution *Robin Youngson*   208

Epilogue Turning the silence into a roar *Soo Downe, Sheena Byrom*   219

Contributors' biographies   222
References   227
Index   251

FOREWORD:
HEARING THE ROAR BEHIND THE SILENCE

Frances Day-Stirk and Sir Sabaratnam Arulkumaran

'There are far too many silent sufferers. Not because they don't yearn to reach out, but because they've tried and found no one who cares.' Richelle E. Goodrich

Silence can mean different things at different times to different people. It can be good; relished by many, craved by others who live amidst the hustle and bustle of their daily lives. There is silence by choice as well as unwanted silence. Silence can be an active energy with the power to get people to think and to act, it can help slow the mind down for quiet reflection. Its importance is also captured in songs like *The Sounds of Silence*.

Who are the 'silent sufferers'? Why do they exist? Of all the definitions of the word silence that speak to silent sufferers it is not 'the absence of sound' or 'a refusal or failure to speak out' which aligns but 'the condition or quality of being or keeping still and silent', which speaks volumes. Throughout the world there are many people who 'suffer in silence'. Included in this group are the silent sufferers in maternity care, both the users and the providers.

This is the subject of *The Roar Behind the Silence* which seeks to raise awareness, explore the causes of distress in maternity care and ways in which we can address the issues, and find solutions – the 'what' and 'how'. This book is welcome. Infused with topics and words such as: relationships, compassion, dignity, kindness, resilience and learning – all key factors. Emphasis is also placed on the importance of the team of providers – midwives, obstetricians and others.

Silence can also be a powerful therapeutic and strategic tool. As Mark Twain, said 'The right word may be effective, but no word was ever as effective as a rightly timed pause'. *The Roar Behind the Silence* sends a message that we are all in it together. And together we can alleviate the distresses. Our challenge is in working together – as service users and service providers – in getting this balance right.

Unlike the introductory quote there are many who care. Some of these voices can be heard loud and clear in the rightly timed *The Roar Behind the Silence*. A welcome and much needed roar. We urge readers to become champions adding voices to this roar. We would do well to be guided by these words of the Dalai Lama '*Love and compassion are necessities, not luxuries. Without them humanity cannot survive*.'

FOREWORD

Toyin Saraki

Having worked closely with midwives through my work with the International Confederation of Midwives, and my organisation, the Wellbeing Foundation Africa, I have been honoured to hear their stories and learn from their experiences. The closer I work with midwives, the stronger my belief that midwives are an integral part of the solution in reducing maternal mortality. The power and perseverance of midwives, and others involved in the safe delivery of newborns, creates an energy that is palpable. This book translates this energy into the written word.

The relationship between a mother and her midwife is rooted in a fundamental sense of mutual understanding and kindness. Caring, respectful and well-educated midwives result in more confident mothers, safer babies, and healthier families with better futures. Bringing together the voices of those committed to safeguarding women and children, Downe and Byrom have provided a platform for a much-needed discussion on respectful and compassionate care. Their goal to change the culture of midwifery from one of fear to one of love is a noble pursuit. After all, love – that echoes the enduring love between mother and child – is a far more compatible emotion for childbirth.

The writers explore how international, national and local systems and models of care can support and empower caregivers and women to engage in healthy, compassionate practices. There is an African proverb that says '*If you want to go fast, go alone. If you want to go far, go together.*' It is in this spirit that we should draw together our voices as women, mothers, midwives and caregivers. Through this collective call we can bring out the best practice and results in childbirth.

I thank Soo Downe and Sheena Byrom for their words, for taking the time to research, and for pulling together expertise from around the world to improve the lives of every woman and every child.

INTRODUCTION:
WHAT'S GOING ON IN MATERNITY CARE?

Sheena Byrom and Soo Downe

As editors of this book, our position is that the issue of kindness and compassion is absolutely fundamental to good quality maternity care. We came to this conclusion as midwives with many years' experience in a range of clinical, research and management roles, working both in and out of hospital settings, and as a consequence of discussions with many people around the world about the state of maternity services. This book is the result of that concern. However, the contributing authors demonstrate that this is a far from simple issue. Many of the chapters offer very specific insights, but there is a recurring factor: fear, and the need to overcome it. In this chapter we summarize the nature and impact of fear as a basis of maternity care and delivery. We have done this to indicate what must be addressed if the maternity services of the future, in all countries of the world, are to deliver optimum care, both for childbearing women and their families, and for the staff attending them. We then complete this opening chapter by outlining the organization of the book, as an overview for the reader.

Fear as a driving principle of maternity care design and delivery

For many years there has been a growing concern about the culture of fear that is penetrating maternity services (Kirkham, 2013; Dahlen, 2014). This work demonstrates that fear felt by maternity care workers is directly and indirectly being transferred to the women and families they serve. For midwives and obstetricians, fear of recrimination, litigation, negative media exposure and loss of livelihood potentially contributes to defensive practice (Symon, 2000). Over-treatment 'just in case' not only increases workload stress and error (Youngson, 2012), but potentially causes iatrogenic damage to mothers and babies (Dahlen *et al*, 2013, Renfrew *et al*, 2014). In maternity services in England, the issue has been exacerbated since the publication of the report from the Mid Staffordshire Trust public enquiry (Francis, 2013), with a subsequent increase in internal and external service reviews and a fear of bad publicity of imposed special measures. Safe and effective health care treatment is the expectation of those receiving care. It is also what most caregivers intend to provide. This is most likely to be evident when relationships can be developed, and when the building of these relationships is in the hands of those who are working together. However, in many settings, the time and autonomy to form such relationships is subject to, and limited by, powerful external controls and barriers. Ballatt and Campling (2011) warn that when control is external it is toxic and doesn't encourage kinship and reciprocity. Over-regulation and control, they believe, feed a culture where those whose intention is kindness and caring are forced to behave defensively.

In a reciprocal vicious circle, response to a growing litigious society has led to increased, organisational risk aversion. Consequently, risk management processes have emerged that increasingly distract health care organizations, and those that work within them, away from the provision of healthcare and towards servicing risk management systems (Ballatt and Campling, 2011). Paradoxically, activities that aspire to improve safety frequently add burden to an already overstretched service, potentially increasing risk. Ballatt and Campling (2011) suggest that a risk averse culture *frequently shows itself to be earnestly filtering the bath water whilst the baby is left to drown*. Whilst Hunter and Warren (2013) found that some midwives in the UK were resilient to these pressures in current maternity services, many are experiencing low morale and burn-out (RCOG, 2011; Birthrights, 2013).

The issues aren't confined to the UK and Europe. There is global pressure on midwives and maternity care workers, due to a rising birth rate in many countries, and increased medical and social complexities of the women using maternity services (Childbirth Connection, 2013; RCM 2013, Renfrew *et al*, 2014; UNFPA, 2014).

At the same time, and potentially as a consequence, accounts of women being afraid of giving birth (Ayers, 2013), and lack of dignity and respect during childbirth are occurring throughout the world (Birthrights, 2013; WRA, 2013). Disrespect and abuse of childbearing women in low and medium resource countries are indirectly impacting negatively on maternal and newborn morbidity and mortality (Bowser and Hill, 2010).

Finding solutions

However, a drive for change is gathering momentum, and there is increasing evidence that kindness, compassion and mutual respect improve efficiency, effectiveness, experience and staff morale (Ballatt and Campling, 2011; Youngson, 2012). This provides hope for the future. But it requires a shift in focus, from a controlling 'tick box' culture to one where kindness and reciprocity is the central driver of healthcare workers and their organizations.

This book is not designed to be an academic examination of these and associated factors, nor is it a 'cook book' of solutions. The style of the chapters ranges from very personal stories using blog-type approaches, to research-based analyses. The intention is to get underneath the headline issues, to find out what is really going on, and to demonstrate how some people have developed and tested ways of changing the risk-averse and fearful orientation of current maternity care services. These changes have taken place in midwifery and obstetric education, in clinical practice, in management, in service user groups, and in social media spaces. Each author provides a summary of their messages and of possible action points for others.

Organisation of the book

The book is divided into three parts.

Part I: Stories and perspectives from maternity care

Maternity workers, as other healthcare professionals, are bombarded with negative stories and reports of when things go wrong. Whilst it is important to acknowledge and learn from human and system failings, there are practice and whole service examples that offer the potential to influence change. In her book McIvor (2013) demonstrates that compassion can be caught not taught, and proposes that the word has to be lived through actions to be meaningful. This notion is evident in this section. The contributing authors have used research, personal stories and anecdotes from practice and experience, to provide inspiration for ways of working that support respectful, compassionate care.

Part II: Principles and theories

There are currently no statistics evaluating shifts towards compassionate and respectful maternity care, and it is an area that has received little attention (Van Lerberghe *et al*, 2014). However, there is evidence that some organizational systems and policies can foster a culture of unkindness, undermining behaviour and bullying which potentially interfere with childbirth processes by negatively influencing those who work in the service and those who use it (Ball *et al*, 2003). The reported consequences are disenfranchised workers, and women who don't access healthcare facilities because they are afraid (Bowser and Hill 2010; Jackson *et al*, 2012).

In order to consider ways to improve kindness and compassion for women using maternity services and those providing care, it's important to explore the principles and theories that underpin and frame current maternity care practice norms, so that alternatives can be proposed and tested. These issues, including the implications for human rights, are explored in this section.

Part III: Making it happen: solutions from around the world

Several chapters in the book describe models of care that the authors believe increase the potential for respectful, compassionate care. This doesn't mean that kind and respectful care isn't possible in other service models, but it demonstrates a correlation between small, midwife-led models built on positive and mutually respectful relationships with obstetricians, service users, and their families, and based in comfortable homely environments with increased satisfaction for both those delivering and receiving maternity care. This offers hope and potential for all maternity services and the inspiring examples within this section offer ideas to enhance the ability to provide compassionate maternity care in all settings.

Conclusion

This book has been written as a resource for all those who provide and commission (purchase) or influence maternity services, globally. The authors include midwives, student midwives, childbearing women, lawyers, doulas, obstetricians, anaesthetists, nurses and maternity care leaders who believe that kindness, compassion and respect are at the core of positive, safer childbirth practices. Throughout the book we have used the term 'maternity care workers' to include the varying members of maternity teams who care for childbearing women throughout the world. Whilst some chapters are specifically written for a particular group of practitioners, or are based in particular countries and/or settings, the key messages are transferable to other professionals. Our intention is to shift the debate and practice of maternity care from being based in *fear* to being based in *love* (*caritas*, the basis of the word 'caring').

Please note: References for this and all other chapters can be found at the end of the book.

PART I

STORIES AND PERSPECTIVES
FROM MATERNITY CARE

1 Putting relationships at the heart of maternity care

Penny Campling

Maternity care is a relational task, and system. The service relies – it could be argued, more than any other – on the relationship between mother and healthcare worker. The utter helplessness of newborn babies, completely unable to survive alone, means that nurturing should be at the heart of the system. A constructive alliance between a caring and attentive midwife or doctor, and a mother who is encouraged to feel an active and respected partner is particularly important. There are also no other areas of healthcare where it is quite so vital to get it right the first time as the process of facilitating the birth of a healthy baby. This mantra from production industry captures the drive for effectiveness, efficiency and safety that has to be the priority for modern obstetric care. Too often, the relational and the 'outcome' aspirations are seen as opposites with advocates polarizing around one or the other perspective. In this chapter, I argue that an intelligent focus on the therapeutic relationship is all-important and can only improve effectiveness and efficiency.

Vicious circles

There is no doubt that many women experience modern obstetric care as a depersonalizing process and that a worrying number of midwives report feeling demoralized. In many developed countries, as law suits against obstetric services increase and the general panic about health services mounts, a vicious circle builds: activities that aspire to improve safety frequently burden an already over-stretched service, potentially increasing risk by introducing ever more distraction, raising anxiety and leaving maternity care workers feeling that they are workers on a production line in danger of losing their professional discernment. In such a toxic environment, altruism can be squeezed out and there is a tendency to feel one is battling against everyone: the doctors, the hospital managers, colleagues on the unit, even the mothers and their partners (who can be seen as potential complainants, and therefore 'the enemy'). But one thing we know for certain about modern healthcare, is that good outcomes depend on good teamwork and on good communication and collaboration between different parts of the system.

An efficient system, quite simply, needs to *bring the best out of everyone involved*. So often in the health service, initiatives aimed at greater efficiency are in truth about a narrow interpretation of accountability –

about documenting information about what one's doing so that others can scrutinize it, rather than actually doing the job better.

The rest of this chapter will explore what *bringing the best out of every-one involved* would look like in practice.

Bringing the best out of the mother

First of all, it is easier to work with mothers who are not too anxious and frightened. High levels of anxiety can have a detrimental effect in so many different ways, including obvious physiological effects on hormones, respiration, blood pressure, pain threshold and brain functioning. A very anxious mother will have a reduced capacity to understand what's going on and what's expected of her and this, in turn, will increase her anxiety, creating a vicious circle.

There is a great deal of research supporting what is in fact common sense: that mothers who have a good relationship with their midwives will have a better experience of childbirth than those who feel they are being processed as if they are on a factory assembly line. Anxiety, in modern society, is usually framed as an individual phenomenon, but in fact is very much influenced by relationships. *Trust* is all-important in the relationship between mother and midwife and will be nurtured by qualities such as attentiveness, kindness and empathic understanding, forming virtuous circles (Ballatt and Campling, 2011). Mothers who trust their midwives will be more easily soothed and reassured. Moreover, research from other areas of healthcare suggest a trusting relationship means patients are more tolerant when things go wrong, and even when mistakes are made, are less likely to make complaints (Minkulince *et al*, 2005).

Bringing the best out of the midwife, doctor, maternity nurse

It is important to ask what sort of qualities maternity care workers would embody in an ideal system (see the Table opposite for a summary). Certainly, we need professionals who have the appropriate knowledge and clinical skills to do the job properly. This means fostering an attitude of constant learning and improvement that goes far beyond ensuring attendance at the requisite mandatory study days. Learning 'on the job' requires highly motivated individuals who take pride in their work, who retain their curiosity about the ever fascinating and complex process of childbirth, and who have the humility and confidence to ask questions – including honest questions about their own practice and how they might have approached a situation differently.

It requires maternity workers who can be thoughtful about the

---

Table: Qualities to nurture in maternity care workers

- Curiosity, a questioning attitude and an openness to new learning.
- The capacity to hold the mother's experience in mind in the face of all that distracts from this.
- An imaginative understanding of how the maternity care worker can make a difference to others' wellbeing and an understanding of how this fits with the bigger picture and other perspectives.
- A confident belief in their own value and the freedom to act to fit the circumstances.
- Insight into the emotional impact of the job and the capacity to contain rather than act out anxiety.

---

mother's experience, and use this understanding to be kind and attentive and remain attuned even when there are lots of competing pressures. This requires the capacity to balance their attitude to technology appropriately, something that gets more and more difficult in the modern clinical environment. It is important to remember that technology is a helpful tool to facilitate our understanding of what's going on and inform our interventions. But tools are to be used and manipulated by us, not the other way round. New technology should be incorporated into our clinical repertoire, enhancing, but never taking the place of, our clinical connection with the patient.

A more malignant cause of distraction away from the childbearing woman can be the increasing bureaucracy that goes hand in hand with the regulatory culture and the competitive market. Much has been written about the unintended consequences of setting targets, for example (Seddon, 2008). Overzealous application and misunderstanding of the place of *evidence-based medicine* has also contributed to increasing levels of bureaucracy with many midwives overwhelmed by guidelines and protocols, lacking confidence in their clinical expertise and unable to pick up when a mother and baby's situation is deteriorating because they are anxiously looking over their shoulder, worrying about following the ever-changing 'rules' and guidelines and stressing over the amount of documentation. The good clinician is one who respects the fact that every individual situation is slightly different. Robots will never be able to deliver babies, and midwives and doctors need to be actively and intelligently balancing on the one hand their clinical wisdom and experience and, on the other, the protocols, guidelines and manuals that are important, but not the be-all-and-end-all of being a professional clinician. The regulatory culture in healthcare can be malignant because, despite the oft-heard moaning that clinical staff spend far too many hours away from the patients filling in forms and filing computer data, the response to every scandal and major untoward incident is to extend regulation, increase bureaucracy and micro-manage staff even further. Good governance requires staff who can balance priorities and are aware of the danger of overloading the system.

Teamwork and collaboration

We need maternity care workers who have an understanding of their role and how this fits with the bigger picture. Often, the hardest thing about this is understanding the role of others in the team – for example, the midwives understanding the doctors and, indeed, the women and families them-selves – and respecting perspectives that are different from their own. At the same time, of course, we need other clinical professionals and child-bearing women – not to mention managers, commissioners, governments and the public at large – to have a better understanding of the role and expertise of midwives in their ability to facilitate normal childbirth. For we need midwives to be more than cogs in the wheel; we need midwives to be grounded in their professionalism, and have a confident sense of their personal agency and freedom to act when this is appropriate.

Ideally, we need all maternity care workers to intuitively monitor their own anxiety levels, and understand what this is telling them about the clinical situation at hand, but not behave in a way that spreads this anxiety into the people around them. Professionals who are unable to contain their own anxiety will find it hard to be sensitive towards their patients' anxiety; in fact, they may well be contributing to escalating anxiety levels, not just in the mother, but in the team around them. Uncontained anxiety is harmful at every level. In addition to high sickness levels, it leads to erratic decision-making and will detrimentally affect outcome, something that was recognized over 50 years ago (Menzies, 1959).

Bringing the best out of the organization

The primary task of managers and leaders at all levels of the organiza-tion is to create the conditions where clinical staff can work at their best. Evidence about what these conditions should be is plentiful and can be drawn from many disciplines including organizational psychology and aspects of management theory, anthropology, social psychology, psycho-analysis and neuroscience (Ballatt and Campling, 2011). Unfortunately, there are many pressures pulling in other directions, but successful ser-vices are those where this task is clearly the priority.

Too often, midwives and doctors see the system as working against them rather than for them. Delivering babies safely is a highly stressful job – emotionally and physically arduous. Midwives, for example, work day in day out with vulnerable, often very frightened women and have to face the reality that things can go badly wrong. The possibilities of death and disablement lurk amidst much joy. Constantly being in touch with such risk is an emotional as well as an intellectual challenge and takes considerable courage.

Midwives and doctors need to be listened to, nurtured, developed and encouraged if they are to enact the qualities required to provide sensitive, compassionate maternity care. Simply put, they will offer a much more effective and caring service if they feel effectively cared for themselves. Perhaps, most important, there needs to be a much better understanding of the emotional task facing those who work in maternity services. This requires managers to make sure there are reflective practice structures in place to help all staff to process the feelings that arise during the course of their work. It also requires managers to be more aware of the way anxiety – in themselves and in those around them – can drive behaviour in unhelpful ways.

Conclusion

The tensions besetting maternity services can feel at times irreconcilable, with morale worsening amongst midwives and doctors. But there is the potential to change for the better if everyone focuses more on relationships and how to bring the best out of the people around them. Maternity care workers who are kind and attentive and better attuned to those in their care, and to their colleagues, are more efficient and more likely to get it right first time. Mothers who feel respectfully attended to are less anxious and better able to be co-operative partners in the birth process. Leaders who dare to insist that their most important task is to care for their frontline staff and ensure that conditions facilitate their clinical work, make a huge difference. If everyone were able to focus just a little bit more on these things, a virtuous circle would be created and there could be a significant shift in the culture for the better.

KEY MESSAGES

- The quality of relationships directly affects care and outcomes.
- A good system brings out the best in everyone involved.
- Modern maternity care depends on good teamwork, good communication and collaboration between different parts of the system.
- Good governance requires staff that can balance priorities and an awareness of the dangers of overloading the system.

ACTION POINTS

- Don't underestimate the emotional task involved in maternity work.
- Make sure you have enough support and a 'safe' forum to process difficult feelings that arise from the work.
- Think carefully about how to sustain yourself in the role and watch out for signs of burn-out.
- Look out for other members of your team, try to sort out conflicts at an early stage and don't let grievances fester!

2 Compassion in hospital care staff: what they think it is, what gets in its way, and how to enhance it

Michael Clift and Senga Steel

Whittington Health is a North London Integrated Care Organization (ICO) consisting of the amalgamation of an acute care trust and two primary care trusts. In the wake of the Francis report (Francis, 2013), like many organizations we were concerned to know how compassionate our organization was, and this chapter describes some of that journey of discovery and highlights our most prominent insights from it.

What we did

Most Monday mornings a team of senior nurses and midwives, who represent the clinical areas in the hospital part of the organization, meets and briefly discusses the pressing issues of the day before the co-ordination of a scheduled audit or survey is carried out by the team. It's called our 'Visible Leadership Programme (VLP)'. The idea is to take the temperature of the organization, to see how healthy it is, to assess the quality of the service and the standards we are achieving. The programme includes assessments of infection control practice, hand hygiene, medicines storage and other pre-planned activities. One of the surveys we carry out is the staff survey and includes simple questions such as, 'Do you like working here?' and the friends and families test, i.e. 'Would you recommend this service to your friends and family?' In response to the Francis Report (Francis, 2013) and the DoH Compassion in Practice recommendations (2012), two compassion-themed questions or prompts to that survey were added which were 'What does compassion mean to you?' and 'Describe an example of where you have shown compassion'.

The responses were collected from the shop floor in brief interviews by the team, or by the members of staff completing paper surveys. We then analysed the 'data' produced by the responses to these two prompts.

However, before doing this we tried to get some idea of how compassion was already defined. At first glance, many definitions of compassion seem to be faith-based, yet, when a Google news analysis of the word 'compassion' was carried out, it transpired that most media descriptions of 'compassionate' behaviour were of a secular origin. The various faiths commonly describe compassion, but we struggled to find a definition created by healthcare staff, who require compassion to respond therapeutically to the needs of their patients (Ballatt and Campling,

2011; Francis, 2013). It then struck us that, as well as providing us with an impression of the values and behaviours of compassion at our own organization, the analysis of the responses given by our frontline healthcare staff could produce a definition of compassion by a multi-faith, multi-cultural workforce that was missing from the wider literature on the subject. This is of particular interest when it is remembered that for centuries, formalized healthcare work was carried out by monotheistic religious orders with their own philosophy of compassion and taken to as a vocation (O'Brien, 2014). The workforce at our organization holds various different beliefs with over half the workforce of an undefined faith or unwilling to disclose it, so there could exist within the workforce different concepts of compassion and how it is carried out.

Two hundred and eighteen responses from a four month period were analyzed thematically by the two authors, who analysed the data separately, in order to reduce bias. The findings were then compared and discussed and found to be largely very similar. We then created a visual model of the collated themes, both large and small, in response to the two questions, producing a model of the concept of compassion and its behaviours (Fig 1). The bigger the 'bubble' the more frontline healthcare staff described that theme. Paler bubbles represent smaller themes that were similar enough to sit within the larger themes found.

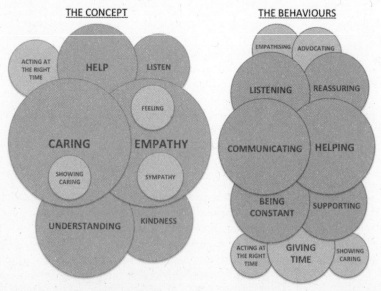

Fig 1: The Compassion Model

What we found

It seemed clear that compassion involved the generation of a feeling as described by words such as 'caring' and 'empathy'. In terms of how this was done, 'communication' and 'helping' were the most common words used. Within both the concept and the behaviours of compassion the theme of time re-occurred. Some staff felt that compassion should be given to all the patients, all the time – 'being constant'. Some staff felt that it was more about seeing when a patient is in distress and acting with compassion at that moment – 'acting at the right time'.

On reviewing the models we had created, we felt the process that was primarily taking place during compassion was one of communication. We then re-arranged our 'bubbles' of themes to represent this process as it took place between staff and patient (Fig 2 and Fig 3).

Compassion begins with an observation, and then communication takes place involving listening and helping. Represented this way, it

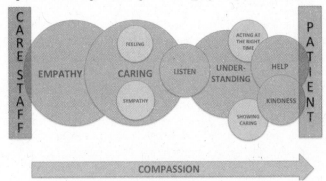

Fig 2: *The Compassion Model – The Concept*

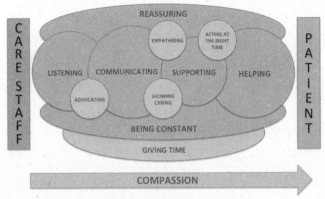

Fig 3: *The Compassion Model – The Behaviours*

became apparent to us that while healthcare work is often broken down into tasks comprised of physical actions, which could be described as 'help', listening is clearly helping too and, done the right way, is a core behaviour of compassion, as regularly described by our own frontline healthcare staff.

The obstacles of compassion

This model was then presented to several focus groups of healthcare staff with the aim of the group to establish what the obstacles to compassion were in terms of showing compassion to patients, and to your colleagues. Several themes emerged which have been represented in Fig 4.

To discuss a selection, 'Technical rationality' relates to the prioritization of technical work and language over care (Kinsella, 2007). The presence of technology within the healthcare environment is significant and those more technical areas of care carry more status. Additionally, it was felt that the presence of technology, such as machines and measuring instruments, acted as a barrier between nurses and patients. 'Judgemental thinking' refers to situations staff described where they would have less compassion for a patient whose lifestyle choices they disagreed with. This situation somehow eroded their ability to feel compassionate and therefore to express compassion through their behaviour. One example given was that of caring for an alcoholic patient with liver damage. Judgements about behaviour and whether a person deserves compassion were a clear obstacle to creating the initial feeling of compassion towards that person's suffering. 'Social environment' refers to the staff support network available in a clinical area. This was usually reflected in support from colleagues, camaraderie, respect for others in the team and good working relationships. This was best illus-

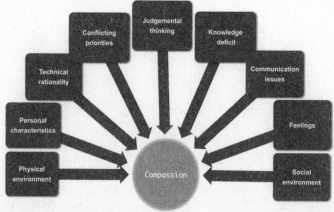

Fig 4: The Obstacles to Compassion

trated by a bank nurse who described attending one area where she was not shown around the ward or told who was in charge and just pointed to the bay where she would be working. She described how this would make her feel withdrawn and less confident and affect her feelings for the patients and staff. This nurse was so hurt by this experience that she became tearful as she related the story. Other nurses described, thematisized under 'conflicting priorities', how when working with temporary staff from the hospital bank or from agencies, those staff were not allowed to do as much (e.g. intravenous antibiotics) so they would have to add that task to their own workload. They also described correcting the 'mistakes' the temporary member of staff had made because they did not know the area and the local processes for getting things done, another addition to their workload. Other staff described how sometimes it was difficult to feel compassion for patients because the patients had withdrawn due to repeated interactions with staff that had lacked compassion because of the various obstacles described. Some staff felt that other staff simply 'didn't have it', that they were not naturally compassionate people. A similar view to that held by Florence Nightingale herself (NMC, 2014).

What do you do about it?

So how do you make staff more compassionate? The obstacles need to be managed and reduced in size and power, and good leadership and management is key here. A feeling of frustration was commonly described in the focus groups, sometimes coming from 'carrying' temporary or weaker staff, to trying to find the right equipment and materials to deliver care. As well as managers working to lessen the external obstacles, staff need to be trained and supported to manage their internal obstacles to compassion in the shape of their thoughts and feelings, such as their frustration in response to external events. This can be done in several ways.

Staff need opportunities to discuss the emotional impact of healthcare in an open and non-judgemental environment. A common question asked at interview is 'How do you know when you are stressed and what do you do about it?' Interviewees often describe variations on 'taking time-out' and in increasingly stretched services managers need to ensure that this opportunity is available, however briefly. Schwartz rounds are a more structured way of taking time-out, where the emotional impact of healthcare is explored using staff stories and case presentations and are increasingly being introduced in UK healthcare organizations. Staff also need to *choose* these more public forums for emotional expression rather than them being mandated. A staff support group within general paediatrics became unpopular (based on survey responses) mainly due to staff feeling 'forced to go'. A monthly session was then introduced where there was an option of discussing distressing cases and their impact, or simply using the opportunity to ask the hospital liaison staff questions to improve their knowledge about various clinical presentations. This group has been much more popular.

Lastly, there are several existing, evidence-based methods of developing greater compassion in healthcare staff of which we will mention three. Compassionate mind training (CMT), acceptance and commitment training (ACT) and kindness behaviour training (KBT). They can all be described as, or influenced by, so-called third-wave therapies, and all involve elements of mindfulness and cognitive behavioural therapy to enhance self-awareness and improve thought and feeling self-management. There will always be internal and external obstacles to compassion but a commitment from each individual in the organization can make a difference to their management and improve the quality of the relationship between staff and patients.

Conclusion

During the analysis of the data it was clear that discussion about compassion takes us to a more humanistic, pre-technical language featuring words like 'caring' and 'kindness' rather than the common shopfloor, task-orientated language of 'medicines' and 'observations'. Within healthcare, the word 'care' seems to have become a word to describe a task that involves a physical intervention from staff to patient, rather than the act of connection and compassion it refers to more commonly in lay language. In the Nursing and Midwifery Council's code of conduct there are 15 mentions of 'care' but none of 'compassion' despite it historically being a core element of care work (O'Brien, 2014). The authors have contributed their findings from this work to the consultation on the 2015 update of the code. It's clear that in the modern, increasingly technical, era of care work we mustn't forget the language and behaviour of our care ancestors and we must re-commit to a core care behaviour of compassion towards our patients and towards our colleagues.

KEY MESSAGES
- Strong leadership means good staff support.
- Supported staff maintain and develop their compassion for service users.
- Consistent teams support each other better.
- Inefficiencies away from the clinical area impact on compassion levels.

ACTION POINTS
- Compassion for service users CAN be maintained and developed.
- Self-awareness and personal resilience are key.
- Take responsibility for your thoughts and feelings.
- Support your colleagues and they will support you.
- Listening IS helping.

3 Dignity in maternity: the power of human rights to improve care for childbearing women

Elizabeth Prochaska

'*Humanity itself is a dignity; for a man cannot be used merely as a means by any man but must always be used as an end.*' Kant, *Metaphysics of Morals*

The principle of human dignity offers a powerful and universal means to improve maternity care. As a guiding value, it enriches relationships between women and caregivers by focusing on basic principles of human worth, autonomy, respect and compassion. As a legal principle enshrined in human rights law, it compels respectful healthcare that takes account of every individual's choices. But despite its potential, dignity is only recently beginning to receive adequate attention in the context of maternity care. This chapter explores the place of dignity and human rights in maternity care and suggests that the transformative power of these principles should be recognized and nurtured by professional caregivers.

A story

We begin with the common story of a mother-to-be, anxiously awaiting the birth of her child, whose pregnancy endures past conventional time limits. Her caregivers tell her she must be induced or her child might die. They do not inform her of the risks to her own body. She suffers a flurry of medical interventions that lead to lasting trauma. The tale is told to emphasize the dangers of over-medicalization and to advocate for gentler birth, but it also teaches us how a mother's interests in childbirth can be treated as secondary to those of her unborn baby. She is given misleading information in order to compel her to sacrifice control over her body to medical professionals. Hospital policies are inflexibly applied. Her care is depersonalized. She becomes a means of production.

How can we help this mother? Traditional resistance to over-medicalization emphasizes that information is power. Women overcome medical hegemony by becoming their own expert through antenatal education. But this model has not stemmed the incidence of unwanted interventions, birth trauma and tokophobia (fear of pregnancy and childbirth). Instead, we need to articulate values before we talk of information and evidence, and we must make women and their caregivers aware of the practical power of those values. The principle of human dignity is the ultimate value on which respectful healthcare depends. It is most powerfully articulated in Kant's categorical imperative: treat a person as an ends and not a means. The relevance of this is immediately apparent in maternity care, when a woman risks being viewed as a means for the creation of life rather than an end in herself. Dignity reinstates the woman as the central agent in childbirth. It demands that her caregivers treat her as a person worthy of respect and capable of making her own autonomous decisions about her child's birth. More than simply avoiding abusive care, the principle of dignity enhances relationships between women and caregivers. A relationship built on respect for the woman's dignity enables each birth to be treated as a sacred event at which the caregivers may share the joy (Matthews and Callister, 2006).

Leave your dignity at the door

Dignity has a good pedigree in bioethics (Foster, 2011). The language of dignity and respect has had a powerful effect on end of life care and has been taken up by organizations campaigning for the rights of the terminally ill (Chochinov *et al*, 2002). Dignity has received less attention in maternity care. The popular saying among pregnant women – 'leave your dignity at the door' – suggests that the birthing room is no place for concerns about modesty or status. In fact, dignity has a pre-eminent place inside the birthing room. In its fullest sense, dignity is a principle that means much more than simple concern for personal status. The imperative to treat a person humanely – as an ends and not a means – protects a person's individual humanity and autonomy.

Research has shown that women's birth experiences are most profoundly shaped by the attitudes of caregivers and women's sense of control during childbirth, the very factors that dignity seeks to promote (Hodnett, 2002; Waldenstrom *et al*, 2004; Stadylmayr *et al*, 2006). The White Ribbon Alliance has recognized the practical power of human rights principles to promote safe maternity care. Their Charter for Respectful Maternity Care, published in 2011, signalled the beginning of a new approach to assessing maternity care that focused on the promotion of values rather than purely clinical outcomes (WRA, 2011).

Caregivers who respect women's dignity protect each individual woman's perception of what it means for her to thrive as a human being. The following account of childbirth is illustrative:

I had my first child in a way I view as traditional, where the doctor was in control and he encouraged me to have an epidural. It was such a frightening experience. Afterwards I thought: 'This isn't childbirth. There's got to be more to it than just lying there with a numb body'.

The woman's description suggests that she believed that there was a way to give birth that would have been consistent with her dignity. For this woman, a dignified birth would have involved active participation (both physical and emotional) in the process and the recognition by her caregivers that she was more than just a 'numb body' (Callister, 1995). The strong theoretical attraction of dignity as a guiding principle is matched by its legal utility. Professional caregivers employed by NHS institutions are under a legal obligation to respect individuals' human rights as set out in the European Convention on Human Rights. The rights in the European Convention were incorporated into UK law in the Human Rights Act 1998, which enables individuals to bring legal claims against public bodies for breaching their human rights. Human rights law – with its foundations in respect for human dignity – provides a powerful corrective to the traditional dominance of clinical negligence law in healthcare. Legal claims for compensation can be made for violation of rights after poor care has occurred, but the real value of dignity exists in its pre-emptive power. When caregivers respect women's dignity, they build a relationship of mutual respect and trust that will guard against harm in childbirth.

Choice and 'risk'

Two examples of issues that commonly arise in maternity care in the United Kingdom are instructive. The first concerns care for women with high Body Mass Index (BMI). Birth centres in the United Kingdom have universally adopted policies excluding women with a BMI over a certain prescribed threshold from accessing their services. Women are told that they are 'high risk' and should give birth on the obstetric ward, where they can be continuously monitored. High BMI policies label women by reference to one, deeply stigmatized facet of their identity, and then apply another label – 'high risk' – that denies them autonomy over their care. If each woman's dignity is to be respected, her caregivers must take fuller account of her as a human being. The law promotes individualized care: it is an unlawful breach of both public law principles and human rights law to apply a policy rigidly without considering making exceptions that reflect a person's individual circumstances.

Many midwives do manage to provide personalized care, even within the culture of risk-management, by planning creatively for women's care, making exceptions to BMI policies or accommodating women's choices within the obstetric ward. This respectful approach to maternity care is greatly assisted by continuity of carer, but it is not dependent upon it. Midwives can support women who seek personalized care by careful antenatal planning in collaboration with a supervisor of midwives.

The second example is maternal request caesarean section. Women who seek a caesarean section without a particular 'clinical' indication are frequently vilified in the media as rich and lazy. In fact, women who choose a caesarean section have often experienced previous traumatic births or suffer a profound fear of childbirth. Their decision to request a caesarean section reflects their autonomous perspective of a good birth. Caregivers have a responsibility to inform women of the risks of the operation, but they should respect that a woman's feelings about birth may differ from their own.

Conclusion

Returning to the mother-to-be, beset by anxiety about her endless pregnancy, dignity gives us the language and the legal framework to remember and respect her humanity. Dignity gives her the courage to demand compassionate care that respects her informed choices, and obliges her caregivers to stand by her as she realizes her own vision of a good birth.

KEY MESSAGES

- The principle of human dignity demands that every person is treated as end in herself and not as a means to an end. It provides a basis for respectful maternity care that treats women as capable of making their own autonomous decisions about birth.
- Human rights law is based on the principle of human dignity. All state healthcare providers, including midwives and doctors, are obliged by the Human Rights Act 1998 to respect the rights set out in the European Convention on Human Rights.
- A human rights approach to healthcare promotes positive and respectful relationships between women and their caregivers that can guard against harm during childbirth.

ACTION POINTS

- Read the White Ribbon Alliance Charter for Respectful Maternity Care.
- Assess your local NHS Trust maternity policies on issues such as induction and access to the birth centre. Do the policies accord with human rights values?
- Observe an interaction between a woman and a midwife and/or doctor during labour. Is she treated humanely and with compassion? Is she given choice about her care and supported if her choice differs from the professional recommendation?
- Consider impediments to respectful maternity care and how these might be overcome.

4 Only for the heartstrong

Olivia Armshaw

As one of the 7243 midwifery students in training in the UK (2012/13) (HoC, 2014), this chapter describes my personal journey into midwifery: through fear, curiosity and wonder; my own birth experience of compassionate midwifery care – to being a student. I reflect on navigating the current landscape of midwifery: its challenges and beauty, and how I feel about the future, including some ways to keep my heart strong, like self-compassion, mindfulness, outdoor swimming and Twitter.

Fear has a lot to answer for

Fear, in a sense, drove me into midwifery: looking for alternatives to the dispiriting brutality and sterility of birth portrayed on TV and the internet, and the infectious tokophobia narrative that seems to drain women's strength and curiosity about our bodies and our selves. While the focus of caregivers appeared to be on trying to eliminate fear; of pain, of losing control, of a bad outcome, I felt that fear was a normal, inevitable part of the experience, that a more useful approach could be to embrace it, creating an environment where feeling afraid or 'losing it' was safe and accepted. Personally, I had experienced birth as a deeply transformative and liberating psychosexual happening, supported by midwives who encouraged me to follow my instincts and have confidence in my body, so I felt safe and unobserved in labour. I know first hand that a well-managed, woman-led birth has the potential to immeasurably enhance a woman's life and sense of herself, heal past trauma on the body, and have lasting positive psychological effects. The converse can also be true: when birth is insensitively managed, clock-watched and interventionist, it can exacerbate existing trauma, or simply feel like medical rape (Kitzinger, 2012)

Approximately 85,000 women are raped on average in England and Wales every year (MoJ, 2013). Since the age of eighteen, when I was raped, I had buried feelings about the event until thirteen years later, when pregnant, I became consumed by an irrepressible rage. Hormones get bad press. They are blamed for women's mood swings, and extreme feelings are often labelled as hysteria. Through my midwifery training I have gained a more accurate view of hormones: that they are highly potent chemicals controlling almost all aspects of our lives, influencing all bodily functions, basic and sublime (Godfrey, 2004). Hormonal changes and the impending transition to motherhood were catalyzing a deep shift in me, and an opportunity for healing. I planned my first birth at home, where I felt safe and in control enough of the environment to fully let go. I saw birth as an extension of my menstrual cycle and sexuality; an instinctive, hormonal process and I wanted it to be an intimate event. The midwife attended in quiet confidence, not dominating, directing or instructing me; but unobtrusively, respectfully keeping watch. When I felt like giving up, instead of: 'no, you can't give up', she listened to me and helped me realize that giving up was not a more comfortable option. My first daughter arrived into the water, as I repeated the word 'release' inside my head. Her birth became the most meaningful experience of my life, and I felt transformed, in awe of my incredible human body. I loved myself. Pregnancy and ultimately birth enabled me to express, release and move on from toxic feelings locked in my body, reclaiming my body with the same intensity as I had lost it. I felt grounded in a deep respect, pride and confidence in my humanness. Through the healing power of birth and good midwifery, I moved on, got free – and found my calling, to boot. I had discovered the potential of pregnancy and birth to affect a woman, and the importance of facilitating it, as far as possible, to occur in a spontaneous unmanaged way, with the hormonal integrity and rhythms intact. I would like to be the kind of midwife who sets the environment for a woman to trust her instincts and have confidence in her body, so she feels safe to express herself freely and does not feel observed. For me, trust is a remedy for fear, and finding ways to engender trust in a woman's own body is a key part of being a midwife – curiosity and wonderment too. It is tragic that women are not curious about our bodies and what we can do; only scared. When I try to unravel the deeper causes of our insecurity, it seems the objectification of female bodies and the sexism inherent in the media representation of women play a part, as well as the routine medicalization of pregnancy and birth.

Spontaneous labour in a normal woman is an event marked by a number of processes so complicated and so perfectly attuned to each other that any interference will only detract from the optimal character. The only thing required from the bystanders is that they show respect for this awe-inspiring process by complying with the first rule of medicine: nil nocere *[do no harm].* Kloosterman, G., Dutch professor of obstetrics, 1982

My own experience of compassionate midwifery care, combined with a yearning for change in public perceptions of birth, and for the sense of wonder described above by Professor Kloosterman – formed the foundation of my student midwife journey. I had done a degree in Human Communication and Social Anthropology twenty years ago, and had worked in Brazil and the UK in a variety of creative and brand copywriting roles, around having my three children. Midwifery is an expression of love and political consciousness, combining health, wellbeing, and the nurturing of women, with human rights and feminism, and is part of women's struggle for equality and control over our own bodies – all in one profession. I never thought the career change would be an easy journey, especially with a young family, but the course is unexpectedly demanding on every level, and transformation into a midwife more profound than I had imagined.

As I morph from third-year student into qualified midwife, I am increasingly concerned about the medicalized, institutionalized and fragmented way women are cared for in the NHS, which feels as if it is being dismantled in front of our eyes. I have had the privilege of working with outstanding mentors, who have naturally modelled compassion, respect and kindness, in a variety of settings: a freestanding midwife-led unit; an alongside birth centre; and a large industrial-sized obstetric unit – amalgamated from two smaller ones – where it sometimes feels that women are processed through labour and postnatal wards, with little time to develop trusting relationships. In early labour many women come into hospital and meet the triage system, not their own trusted midwife. Although we can work openheartedly to build rapport and trust quickly, it can feel like the best of a bad job, because we know that women have better birth outcomes with a known and trusted midwife (Sandall *et al*, 2013). The postnatal care situation is particularly worrying and I do not know how to give women the time and care they need, especially breast-feeding support, when there is such rapid turnover on the busy wards. The system seems broken and I feel powerless to fix it. I am profoundly grateful for my placements at the freestanding midwife-led birth unit in the heart of the community – which also has a 5% home birth rate (double the national average), where midwives work extremely hard to provide continuity of carer. These community experiences of getting to know women throughout their pregnancies have given me a feeling of true midwifery, and I am excited about caseloading women in this final year of training.

The report on the Mid Staffordshire NHS Foundation Trust Inquiry (Francis, 2013), which highlighted a shocking need to change our healthcare system, affected morale across the UK. For me this was compounded by a heart-wrenching article in the *Independent* (2014) by an anonymous midwife outlining her reasons for resigning, after a decade, from the job she loved. It could have been written by any number of midwives I know, who are frustrated and demoralized; who feel they cannot use their skills, but do not want to act as obstetric technicians (Ball, Curtis and Kirkham, 2002); or who are exhausted by what feels like dangerous skeleton staffing, the rise in the birth rate, the increasing complexity of pregnancies and social factors, and the lack of midwives to share the workload. The article shook me surprisingly deeply, making me question my commitment, the strength of my compassion, level of resilience, depth of my love, and the impact on my family – oh the irony of helping women transition to motherhood whilst reneging on my motherly duties!

I feel sad that genuine choice of care and place of care is not uniformly available across the UK, or indeed the world. In 2014 the future of independent midwifery swung precariously in the balance as lack of accessible affordable insurance for independent midwives meant they might be forced into extinction. On a bitter March morning we students, haggard from night shifts and travel to London, marched on Downing Street like suffragettes, with 'affordable insurance' placards, along with independent midwives, NHS midwives, doulas, mothers, fathers and children. Thanks to the tireless *Save Independent Midwives* campaign, a workable solution has been found and for now the way seems clear, so choice – albeit at a price – is safe.

On placement, it is my mission to find midwives who profess that, even knowing what they know now, would still choose to be a midwife; those that love it and would not rather do anything else, are solid gold and I magnetize towards them. At a hospital antenatal unit I attended on placement, I absorbed as much as I could from the lovely midwives there, who make every effort not to pathologize women, looking instead for ways to make things cosy and unmedicalized – they are so kind and just plain nice to the women. What struck me was their lack of differentiation between the women and each other, the midwives, doctors and students – just an air of respect and compassion for all: ensuring everyone had proper, timely lunch breaks and left work on time; making rounds of tea for each other; sharing the boring admin jobs; having a laugh even when clinics were overflowing, and no talk of blame. The unit manager is shiningly kind and I felt nurtured and cared for there.

In my final year of training, thanks to Iolanthe Midwifery Trust, I did an elective midwifery placement at Hospital Sofia Feldman in Brazil, an oasis of humanized care in an extremely medicalized birth culture: national caesarean rate of 50.1% (Leal, 2012); syntocinon drip and amniotomy used on 40% women; 91.7% of vaginal births are in lithotomy; 36.1% with uterine fundal pressure; 53.5% episiotomy (Leal, 2014), and

65.2% without birth partner during labour (Diniz *et al*, 2014). However humanization – synonymous with the *Dignity in Childbirth* and *Respectful Maternity Care* agendas (Birthrights, 2013; White Ribbon Alliance, 2011) – is gaining momentum, and Brazil, once famous for its high caesarean section rate, is now becoming known as the place where change is happening. Humanization is not just about lowering the intervention rate, but the simple addition of kindness, compassion and respect to our work, shown through eye contact, smiling, holding a hand, explaining and discussing options clearly, appropriately exploring consent, and including birth partners. These simple behavioural habits are how we make a difference wherever we are, yet I have noticed that when the pressure is on, they can be the first elements of care to disappear. I learnt so much from the Brazilians who are committed to supporting women to birth their babies in a gentle, physiology-enhancing environment; fighting to strengthen midwifery and end obstetric violence of all kinds. And although more extreme in Brazil, the principles of humanization are just as relevant in the NHS Trust where I work.

I feel like I am coming into midwifery with my eyes opened to a fairly bleak landscape in which midwives are longing to give the compassionate care we are trained for, despite the many factors blocking our way. The pockets of loveliness, shining midwives, movements for Normal, Better and Positive Birth; for human rights in childbirth, to save independent midwifery, and to embed the 6Cs into maternity services (Care, Compassion, Competence, Communication, Courage and Commitment) (DoH, 2013) – are all testimony to this longing, and I feel optimistic about the future. Mostly. I am concerned about how I will manage to uphold my ideals of compassionate care, keep the love flowing, build my own resilience, wellbeing and positivity, and not burn out.

I find solace and wisdom in Gilbert's *The Compassionate Mind* (2009), which links self-kindness and self-compassion with well being and coping with stress. In the section on building the compassionate self, he cites mindfulness as the first step, that is, learning how to pay attention in the present moment without judgment. It is a way of understanding 'attention' and choosing to direct it to a particular experience or sensation – being in the moment (Gilbert, 2009).

After completing a mindfulness-based stress reduction course, I try to be mindful in practice, sometimes doing the three-minute breathing space in the toilet: a mini-meditation that can be used anywhere when things feel overwhelming or difficult, to feel grounded in the present moment again. It is a process of becoming more conscious – by noticing and acknowledging what is there in me, what is going on for me, what I am feeling, I am better able to be present to others, specifically who I am caring for. Beddoe and Murphy's (2004) study of an eight-week mindfulness-based stress reduction course for nurses showed that their mindfulness practice facilitated empathic attitudes, as well as decreased their tendency to take on others' negative emotions. Shapiro (2005) suggests the added bonus that such self-care trickles down to improve the quality of the therapeutic relationship.

Self-care is paramount. This is not just about taking breaks, keeping hydrated and having a laugh at work – but outside midwifery, it is essential to prioritize swimming; sleep; good food; time with my family, and friends if I am lucky. These things are not just 'nice to have', they are part of my survival kit and when I do not make time for them, I am much more vulnerable to mental and physical problems. I cannot be an authentically compassionate, energized midwife if I am exhausted, hungry, uncomfortable and stressed. Professor of human development and self-compassion expert, Dr Neff (2011) recommends that at any moment you feel challenged beyond your ability to cope, try giving yourself compassion, which might involve putting your hand on your heart to physically comfort yourself and say something nurturing and supportive to yourself (as you would to a close friend).

Last but not least: Twitter, the great community builder and network maker, has helped me grow as a student midwife, nurtured, sustained and educated by connections and relationships. I have become part of a 21st century feminism; social media enabling faster and wider sharing of activism, experiences, ideas, schemes, policies, events, and conferences. Twitter is a forum for debating and promoting issues: normality in childbirth, human rights in maternity care, reducing fear, the patriarchy, failings of institutionalised postnatal care, to name but a few. It provides a means to conserve energy and thrive, helping me balance these bigger questions with my everyday interactions of care. I found my Twitter voice engaging in meaningful conversations with students, midwives, midwifery elders, obstetricians, researchers, doulas, campaigners and healthcare practitioners. I have challenged and been challenged – silenced even, and discovered new people to love, learn from, and admire. The nourishing ecosystem on Twitter is helping me develop as a post-modern midwife, globally conscious and connected (Davis-Floyd, 2007).

Our birth culture is driven by fear and blame, and I admit it: I am afraid of making serious mistakes; causing harm inadvertently; missing something important – not to mention the ever present spectre of litigation and loss of professional registration, before I have even achieved it. I hope that when I qualify I will be supported with a preceptorship, not left alone to deal with complex situations too soon. I hope that delivery suites will look like birth centres. I hope that postnatal care becomes valued so we have time to care. I hope more women choose to birth at home. I hope for more midwives. I hope I can keep my heart strong. I owe it to myself, my three daughters and their daughters, to generate a renewed trust and curiosity in our bodies, and respect and compassion for childbearing women, and midwives (ARM, 2013).

KEY MESSAGES

- Compassion plays an essential part in woman-led care, which can enhance a woman's life and sense of herself, and have lasting positive psychological effects.
- Concern about a medicalized, institutionalized and fragmented maternity care system being inconducive to compassion, kindness and respect, as women feel processed through the busy wards, with little time to build relationships with midwives.
- Committed, determined midwives strive extremely hard to provide the care we are trained to give, in spite of exhaustion, dangerous staffing levels, fear of litigation, low morale and pay freeze. But at what cost to ourselves, our health?
- Cause for optimism: the strength and love of midwives; the movements for Normal, Better and Positive Birth; for human rights in childbirth, to save independent midwifery, and to embed the 6Cs into maternity services (Care, Compassion, Competence, Communication, Courage and Commitment).

ACTION POINTS

- Consider using mindfulness as a way to help yourself, and others.
- Join Twitter and start connecting with the global midwifery network.
- Prioritize self-care: sleep, balance with family life, exercise, and nourishing healthy food.
- Become a notes ninja: paperwork and computing are only going to increase, so if we students and new midwives focus on becoming speedy, accurate and subtle – so women don't feel it's our main focus – then we will have more time to be with the women.
- Be compassionate to yourself.

5 When silence roars: Finley's stillbirth

Mel Scott

Maternity service staff are in a position to have a really important impact on the lives of the people in their care. Compassionate, individualized, responsive care has the power to change the way an event is experienced. This is never more true than with families who experience the death of a baby. Here, I describe the birth (and death) of my son Finley, highlighting the importance of the care I received. I am passionate about the difference that kindness and compassionate care can, and does make in maternity services. This is my story.

Being pregnant, giving birth

In 2008 I discovered that I was pregnant. Sadly, this pregnancy ended with a roller coaster of tests with each little glimmer of hope gradually taken away, until we finally realized that we were going to lose our baby at eight weeks. Strangely, this loss cemented my desire to become a mum and six months later I was pregnant again. After a quiet first trimester, I settled into pregnancy happily. It never even occurred to me that anything could happen at the other end of pregnancy. I prepared for a natural, water birth with hypnotherapy, reiki, reflexology and took care of myself well. Our lovely community midwife was so supportive, never once questioning any of my wishes. Finally at 41+5 I thought my waters had broken so we went to hospital.

I arrived at the birthing unit at 10.30pm and at that point things stopped following my well-laid plans. There was meconium in my waters, so it was explained that I would not be able to have a water birth and I was asked about induction which I declined. I was assessed on the labour ward, and reassured that, as I was not yet dilated or contracting, I would be admitted to the antenatal ward and have monitoring every four hours. My husband was sent home.

I sat alone listening to my hypnotherapy CD, and a couple of hours later got increasingly more worried that I had not felt my baby move and that the meconium had got thicker and darker. I asked to return to the monitor and noticed that my baby's heart rate was dropping. I called the midwife to look, and each of the three times this happened, I was reassured that there was an explanation. Eventually, she stayed to watch and saw the heart rate drop herself. A doctor arrived at which point the heart rate dropped again. The doctor decided to do an ultrasound, which showed a present, but slow, heart beat. The senior midwife at this point encouraged an emergency caesarean. My last memory of my pregnancy is of a tear rolling down my cheek, and the smell of rubber as the mask was pushed onto my face.

My boy

At 6.13am Finley John Scott was born without a heart beat. He didn't wake up.

I awoke to the news that I had a son, but that he hadn't made it. My husband and parents arrived at the hospital to find out that I had had surgery and that Finley had died.

My life changed that day. It was never going to be the life I had planned. In an instant my dreams were taken away from me. And yet we would never return to the life that was either. We were lost. I have very few memories of my own from the first day. I was confused and sleepy, recovering from anaesthetic and morphine. While I was asleep, the midwife helped my husband to bathe Finley. This time was videoed for us. The midwife was so gentle, handling Finley just as she would any newborn baby, kindly explaining how to wash him.

My mum asked me if I wanted to hold my son. I didn't want to. She gently handed him to me, and I began to realize that I had become a mum. Some photographs were taken, including a family photograph capturing the moment that two became three. Finley had his hand and footprints taken too. As the hours passed I began to get to know my son. I gently stroked the fluffy blanket and soon wanted to hold him, and never to let him go. The midwives did not mind me calling them to hold him while I used the bathroom. They understood I did not want him left alone and cold.

The night after Finley was born each of the staff that worked in the theatre came to see me. Without exception, they all cried with me. The anaesthetist, the doctor, they both were so sorry for what had happened. I am so grateful that they came to acknowledge what had happened. That was the first time that I realized this tragedy had affected everybody.

The bereavement midwife was fantastic. She helped us to understand that we had to capture a lifetime of memories in a few short moments. We have clay footprints, photographs of Finley in different outfits, video footage of his blessing with the chaplain. Friends and family visited and the midwife gently explained to each one that we had Finley with us, and that we were holding him. They explained to use his name and refer to him in the present tense, which helped us come to terms with what had happened in our own time.

In all we spent three days in hospital and Finley stayed with us the whole time. We did not experience anything except kindness and compassion. Even the topic of going home was broached gently by the bereavement midwife. She came to see me before her shift ended – and stayed long past the time she should have left. She suggested taking some photographs and captured some beautiful, tender images – even suggesting that I kiss my son (which I had not known I was allowed to do). She gently explained that I would need to leave hospital the next day, and asked what I would like my last memory of Finley to be. She sat quietly as I sobbed that I had not even changed my son's nappy.

She showed no judgement just wrote down my wishes to undress my son, change him, bathe him and get him ready for bed. She agreed to communicate this to staff on duty the next day, and helped me decide that I wanted to leave Finley with a midwife, in the room we'd stayed in, while we left.

This gentle, compassionate, empowering approach enabled me to plan the most difficult thing I have ever had to do. It gave me choice, where I felt that I had none. My choices were respected, even the unusual request to bathe him three days after his death. My husband recorded those moments, as I bathed and dressed my son for the first and only time, cradled him in his pyjamas and read him a bedtime story. I left hospital, broken and empty but without anger. I left hospital feeling well cared for and supported.

Finding out

It was much later that other people began expressing their concerns about our care during labour and it began to occur to us that something had gone horribly wrong. I wrote a list of questions for our appointment with the bereavement midwife, but she was unable to help answer some of them as she had not been present during labour. The second opportunity for us to find out what had happened was presented when we went to find out the results of the post-mortem.

This was my first experience of a lack of compassion and understanding. As we sat in the maternity waiting room waiting to hear what had killed our baby, all I could see was walls filled with beautiful black and white images of newborn babies. I counted nine bumps and so many smiley faces. We received the results in an office surrounded by three breastfeeding posters, numerous birthing books and the noise of crying babies. The post-mortem was inconclusive, but again the opportunity to tell us, with honesty, that things could have been improved, was missed.

We felt that we weren't being listened to. We'd been continuously told that what happened to Finley happened quickly, and was unpreventable. But I could not understand this.

We decided, against my better judgement, to appoint a solicitor. I was concerned about the impact of this process on me. I was right to be concerned.

Over a four-year period I would find out every little detail about my labour, including a suspicious heart trace that was not noticed or acted upon correctly on my arrival at the hospital, and a mention of my choice not to be induced changing the appropriate course of action and impacting the decision not to admit to labour ward. I had gone from blaming nobody to blaming myself, and the staff involved. I would also learn of the 30-minute delay in getting the doctor, and that some of the decisions could have been made in a different way. I found myself in the unbearable position of holding knowledge about mistakes in my care but not being able to act upon them legally because no expert would state that they were more than 61% sure that Finley would have survived if everything that could have been done, was done.

I asked for advice and was told that we could report the midwife to the Nursing and Midwifery Council, and the doctor to the General Medical Council. I didn't want this. It would do nothing except adding stress to those people who looked after us, perhaps losing one more good midwife from the profession. All I wanted was for someone to tell me the truth, and say they were sorry and to take steps to make sure it didn't happen again. Nothing anyone does can change the situation. My son is dead and will remain dead. It hurts every single day, but what hurt more was that people would not tell us what had really happened.

The truth

Almost five years after Finley was born, I met with the head of midwifery. She looked through my notes. I sent her the reports that we had received. I went with an open mind, not knowing what to expect, but knowing that I had some suggestions to make. Within minutes of being there she explained that she agreed with the reports, that some of the care that we had received and decisions that had been made could have been improved, and perhaps that the caesarean could have been done earlier. We reached the same place of understanding, which is that we will never know what difference that improved care could have made. I feel no need to try to prove he would have survived. He didn't. The process of trying to prove that someone is to blame is too hard. I can't face it.

I am pleased to hear that some changes had already been made to processes. There is now the opportunity to call back staff from the community at busy times, or ultimately to shut the unit if it is unsafe to remain open to new admissions.

My concerns were listened to, for example that I had a combination of risk factors which were not considered together. They also considered acting upon some of my suggestions such as to offer parents a room to meet away from the maternity reception and labour ward when getting postmortem results and for all stillbirths/sudden deaths to be acknowledged by the hospital with a simple, compassionate letter saying they are sorry for the family's loss. Most importantly we will work together to transform Finley's birth story into a case study from which other staff can learn.

If you look only at the statistics, the opportunity to make a difference to the family is lost. I am one of many statistics. I am one of 11 families in the UK every day who experience stillbirth, 4,000 a year. It sounds a lot. Not if you look at an alternative statistic. I am also the 4.9 in 1,000 births – but that makes me sound rare. Up to 30% of stillbirths are thought to be preventable – yet we have not reduced this rate significantly in the last decade.

A few years ago I began to wish there was another way. A way that doesn't involve anger and fear, blame or more pain. A way that shares the truth, from a place of compassion and allows the lessons that need to be learnt, to be learnt nationwide. I found another way.

Conclusion

If we look at the story behind the statistics, the emotional impact, the ripples affected by everyone, the support costs, the impact on employment, and the personal toll of stillbirth, we will see that even one death is too many. Compassionate care takes the personal story into account – and helps ease the effects of the devastation. It was a very long time before I felt anger about what happened during my labour and birth. This was largely due to the excellent bereavement care we received. Never underestimate the power of time, compassion and communication in moving towards a place of peace and healing.

True compassion holds honesty as a value. It is unfair to subject parents to many years of investigations, reports and heartache. Perhaps by examining with openness each difficult situation – and openly discussing the findings with parents, lessons can be learnt in a timely manner. If the philosophy openly changed to show these lessons learnt – preferably the first time something happens, not after repeated occurrences, it would ease the feeling that nothing ever changes. It feels so helpless to look at the sad situations that occur and think that there is no way to change things. It must also inspire helplessness in staff. There is something empowering and supportive in exploring the learning points from tragic situations, near misses but also from situations that work well.

My story highlights the positive impact that adequate, skilled support after loss can bring. Sadly, this support is not always available to every parent, in every hospital around the country. In the course of my work, I have become aware that there is little support for maternity staff following caring for a family who experience a death. It is important to recognize that there is an impact upon staff, and provide support to individuals and staff teams following distressing situations, enabling them to continue with their work.

Kindness and compassion matter to us all.

KEY MESSAGES

- Value the story behind the statistics. If we look at the personal toll of stillbirth, we will see that even one death is too many. Compassionate care takes the personal story into account – and helps ease the effects of the devastation.
- Organizational honesty eases self-blame. True compassion holds honesty as a value. It is unfair to subject parents to many years of investigations, reports and heartache.
- Many parents just want answers, want to understand and most of all for it not to happen again. There is no need for this process to be a lengthy legal one.
- Compassionate (bereavement) care diffuses anger.
- Change the focus from one of accusation, blame and cover up to one of lessons learnt – no matter how tough those lessons are. There is an opportunity for learning in every situation.
- Provision of support for staff and parents after loss is crucial.

ACTION POINTS

- Remember the power of time, compassion and communication in moving towards a place of peace and healing.
- Be open and honest, whatever the consequences.
- Listen to those you care for. Compassionate care takes stories into account.
- Learn from mistakes.

6 Birth thoughts from Hungary: eternal gratitude

Anna Ternovszky

Mothers' birth stories are important. They help us to understand what matters at the most vulnerable yet potentially most powerful time of a woman's life. Stories that include conflict with maternity systems bring the reader to a different point, if the voice is heard. Anna's birth story is not unique – it is repeated every minute of every day, in every country in the world. But the birth of Anna's second baby is significant in that it made international headlines, due to her determination to apply to a court of law to 'allow' her to have a home birth. Anna did this because she believed she would receive more kindness and compassion having her baby at home, in Hungary. In Anna's world, this was the safest thing to do. Now let's hear why.

My choice

Well, I am a mother who decided to give birth to my two little boys at home, surrounded by my family, my loved ones and the midwives and doulas of my choice. It was the best choice I have made in my life. Their deliveries are my most precious memories, something I will always treasure. And I will forever be grateful to those who were by my side at that time, helping me with love and devotion, caring about nothing else but me and my babies.

At the age of 23 – when my first baby was conceived – I asked all my friends who had already had a child, what it was like to give birth. Those – with a few exceptions – who had delivered their babies in hospital, had terrible, sad, traumatic stories to tell me. Those who had given birth at home were all talking with a big smile about it as the happiest time in their lives. So I decided to have my first boy delivered at home. The mandatory prenatal care made me even more opposed to choosing the hospital. They told me that, due to my baby's head diameter, a caesarean section would surely be necessary. I made the right decision. I gave birth at home to both my children without needing this intervention. Feeling safe and secure, to me, meant being at home in those situations, surrounded by the well-known scents and lights that are part of my everyday life, having the loving presence of my husband, my siblings and friends, as well as the support of my midwives and doulas.

Happiness, freedom, love, respect

What comes to my mind when I think of giving birth? Happiness, free-

dom, love, respect, peace, trust, security, self-confidence, being supported and so many other merely positive words. How do I remember it? It
was dawn on a beautiful summer's day when it all started. Early morning,
with contractions seven minutes apart, I went to the Khrishna temple to
dance, then I took the dog out to the woods for a long walk. After that I
returned home to let myself deeply engage with the oncoming experience. Slowly, everyone I hoped to be around me arrived. My husband, my
twin sister, my two midwives, my doula, two friends and my dog. This
was just perfect; I was missing nobody else.

And nobody was too much. There is no way that I would be allowed to
be surrounded by so many people in any of the hospitals. And from that
moment on it was all about me. They were watching all my movements,
my sighs, in complete silence with full attention. One of them was helping
me drink with a straw until the sun came up next morning, the other
was putting hot fermentation on me, one comforted me when I vomited,
another massaged me. When one of them got tired, they just took turns.
Everyone knew what his or her task was to help me best, in silence. I was
gaining so much power and self-trust from the love radiating from them,
and the unwavering faith in my ability to give birth on my own. When I
felt like I was within an inch of death, and all I wanted was for my life to
end, they still believed, and it gave me further strength from contraction
to contraction. They would let me do whatever I wanted to. I was sitting
in the hot bath for over ten hours, pouring hot water on my stomach
during my contractions. I was probably angry with them at times, but
they just looked back with full love in their eyes.

Loving attention

My midwife, Ágnes Geréb, to whom I am most grateful, never left me
for a second. She sat next to me letting me scream, bite her, and throw
pillows at her, yet she always looked at me with the greatest affection and
encouraged me with loving eyes, not shaming me for a moment. I could
be totally myself. Unscrupulously. The constant loving attention gave me
security, and strength all along. To be a woman is special quality. The
midwives were the ones who really knew what I was going through and
felt for me. They treated me like a goddess and with their help giving
birth was the most amazing experience.

I could do whatever I wanted, even if I had never done it before. I
was given an opportunity to have a real meeting with myself and
experience the immense power that lies within me. To this day it gives
me great strength to recall and build upon that feeling. By being able
to focus inward, I was also allowed to pay attention and feel how I was

working in sync with my baby. I felt how we fought as a team; when my uterus contracted, and my baby gathered all his strength, pushing his way outward, I could feel his every movement, and it was simply the most amazing co-operation between the two of us. The love that surrounded me as I was pushing him out was also something I will never forget; my sister and my doula were kneeling face to face, and their legs formed a living birth chair.

With my second boy I couldn't decide whether I wanted a quick and easy birth or if I would prefer a good, long and painful delivery just so that I could enjoy the process as much as possible. I am so glad that it turned out to be a long labour. And I was even more secure because I knew what I was going through, and that all my loved ones and helpers were there with me, so I was sure to make it. Again, I sat for hours in the bath, I got a hot fermentation on my stomach and my waist, massaging my cervix with warm oil, and gave me water to drink... the good well-known security. My wonderful midwife, Ágnes, kneeled on the rough stone floor massaging my back, singing and giving me compresses, holding my hand tight whenever I asked. I did not feel uncomfortable for a second, not even when I was on my hands and knees, yowling and writhing completely naked. I did not have to 'behave', nobody said anything – I felt accepted. As I was shouting that I couldn't go on, Ágnes should do something, she just smiled at me, put my hand on my vagina and said to me:

'Do you feel it? It is your baby's head. He will be born very soon.'

And I was squatting, holding his head in my hand, as he came in to this world. I immediately put him on my heart, and soon afterwards started breastfeeding him. We remained immersed in one another for days. They washed my baby with loving care but never took him away from me. They waited until the umbilical cord had stopped pulsating, and then let his father cut it.

Conclusion

I truly wish that humanity might believe again that women are capable of giving birth the way they want to, and trust in us. I wish women could be themselves in the hospitals, as well, and get the 100% affectionate loving care they deserve in these few hours. I wish that more and more women could tell the story of their giving birth as a wonderful experience rather than a serious trauma for a lifetime.

With both babies, I held them immediately close to my body, and breastfed them. I try to imagine what it is like for a baby to leave the safety of his or her mother's womb and arrive in this unknown world. How scary and painful the journey must be in and of itself, and when he or she arrives and takes those first gasps for air, everything is new. The temperature changes and the sharp light in the eyes must be devastating. The only thing that remains the same is the baby's mother. The familiar rhythm of her heartbeat, the warmth of her body, her voice; the only safe place is with her. That is why I felt that it was crucial for my baby to stay with me upon his birth; something that is allowed in some cases in hospitals, yet which is unfortunately prohibited in many situations.

I am proud of my children, my husband, my sisters, my midwives, my doulas, my friends, and last but not least of myself, that we were able to work together so that I was able to give birth to my children there and then as I wanted, and as they wanted to be born.

Eternal gratitude.

KEY MESSAGES

- When giving birth childbearing women should have the birth supporters they want with them, and should be free to do what they want.
- Mothers' birth stories are important.
- Women deserve 100% respectful loving care when they give birth in hospital, as well as at home.
- Positive birth stories need to be told; we only seem to hear traumatic ones.
- Wherever possible, babies and mothers should not be separated after the birth.

ACTION POINTS

- Love, or at least full respect, works both ways.
- 100% listening to my needs or wishes (massage, compress, silence, hug, drink, vomit, cry, eat...)
- It was the most beautiful feeling during my labours, that I was at the centre of everybody's focus. It was my special time, and all of their energy served only to fulfil my desires with love.
- Help me feel comfortable in any situation and not feel embarrassed if I am naked, scream or poop....
- And trust each other. I need to feel that I have faith in the professional judgement of my midwife, and that I can trust her advice.

7 Don't forget Dad! How does treating dads compassionately fit in with woman-centred care?

Dean Beaumont

Woman-centred care during pregnancy and birth is something which many are thankfully now striving to make a reality. The idea that the woman is at the heart of all decisions about her care, taking her as an individual rather than part of a series of routine processes, is long overdue.

However, when working towards true woman-centred care, I frequently come across the opinion that with limited time and resources it is important to focus energies around education and support solely for the mother, as it is this which is crucial. When I ask about fathers, I am informed that they are 'of course important' but with limited resources, not an essential part of making woman-centred care a reality. My work with dads has often been viewed as a nice optional 'extra' rather than of making any critical difference, with little understanding of the implications for women. This perhaps is not unexpected, given that even the NICE guideline 'Routine care for the healthy pregnant woman' (NICE, 2008) spends 56 pages discussing woman-centred care, without once mentioning fathers.

To me, woman-centred care, or any other phrase we choose to use to describe empowering maternity care, should mean the following: 'To provide accessible and unbiased information and support, empowering the woman to make informed choices about all aspects of her pregnancy and birth.'

A very simple statement and mostly self-explanatory. However, when considering the 'support' being provided to the woman concerned, this has to consider the role of ALL those key support persons for the mother during her pregnancy and birth.

Person-centred practices have been promoted for many years across different health and social care arenas, and one of the key features of any such practice is about creating a circle of support around the individual to achieve their wishes and goals. Specific, named individuals who take responsibility to support the choices of the person are at the centre of the care plan. Transposing this concept to the idea of a woman-centred care plan for pregnancy and birth, there are many professionals who obviously could hold a key role here, such as a midwife, health visitor, doctor, etc. However, for any woman who is in a relationship with the father of her baby, he must be seen as a critical part of this support circle too. Indeed, his influence can be immense – not least because he is also the one person in the support circle who will still be there when many of the professionals have handed over their responsibility – his role as a father, partner/husband and support person, hopefully continues on.

With this in mind, I ask one question: What is the potential if he was equipped with the confidence and knowledge to really support his partner with her wishes?

The influence of dad (the father)

Health professionals do some amazing work. Striving to encourage fathers to act as a better support mechanism does in no way serve to detract from that or undermine this. But it is also essential to note that the impact of the actions and opinions of fathers cannot be underestimated. How many women have said *'I would love to have a home birth but my husband isn't comfortable with it'* and because they are a partnership and she cares about his opinion, she opts for a hospital birth instead? This is a clear instance of where working with the father can potentially open up the choices available to the woman further – I have seen many examples of this with dads attending the groups I facilitate. Once the fathers learn about the birth environment and the role of a midwife in a way which makes sense to them, they leave motivated and enthusiastic to discuss all the options with their partner. What a fantastic way of empowering a woman to feel she really does have access to a wide range of birth choices, by empowering fathers to feel they do have a role in exploring the options with their partners, and feeling confident in supporting her preferences!

This influence of men on decision-making and outcomes does not just extend to birth. Consider breastfeeding for a moment. There are still a number of breastfeeding antenatal classes taking place nationally and globally, which are for women only. This is despite the numerous studies (too many to list here without becoming cumbersome) which evidence how crucial the beliefs of the father are to the initiation and continuation of breastfeeding. Indeed, one study (Wolfberg *et al,* 2014) used a two-hour antenatal session with fathers, consisting of infant care information as well as encouragement for fathers to advocate for breastfeeding and assist their partners. The results were 74% breastfeeding initiation among the women whose partners had attended the class, compared to 41% in the control group. In another study (Cohen *et al,* 2004) in America, a programme offered fathers the opportunity to attend a men-only antenatal session and a one-hour, individual coaching session about breastfeeding. For the fathers who attended both the results were higher than average breastfeeding rates – 69% of their partners were still feeding at six months, compared with the national average of 21%. Now if a woman wishes to attend a breastfeeding class on her own, that would of course be her choice. However, if a woman's goal is to breastfeed and the only option is a class for women only, then are we really supporting her goals, when we don't recognize the importance of the education of the father in that goal as shown by the evidence?

'Typical' dads

Social norms have changed a lot over relatively recent years, and it is now commonplace for fathers to be present at the birth of their child, and also with improvements in paternity allowances in some countries, for them to be at home with their partners for the first early weeks. Some men *are* more anxious about their role in an arena which is unfamiliar to them, especially if they have not been attending regular antenatal appointments with their partners. Men are emotionally usually a little way behind their partners during pregnancy, and one report even suggested *'fathers may not feel their relationship with the baby starts until they are 6 months old'* (DoH, 2011). This could be the result of men feeling like they don't belong, or that it's expected of them to return to work, which can result in a disconnect between mum, dad and baby. This can also be the result of attitudes of professionals who have not considered the harm which their comments might make, or who indeed just show a lack of understanding and compassion.

Words matter

I've been on many maternity unit 'tours' where I have heard a midwife jokingly tell dads off in advance about 'not putting on the TV' or 'not sitting playing games on your phone' – talking to the dads on the tour as though they are naughty children who will need to be handled while their partner is busy giving birth. While there might be an important message here, the way it is delivered can be either empowering or patronizing. Certainly delivered in this way, it is not compassionate or respectful of the enormous journey and possible emotions they may be internally dealing with. The reality is that some men will do these things, but more often out of a lack of understanding of what they could be doing, rather than because they do not care. Nervousness kicks in when men feel helpless and like 'a spare part', and they potentially do these things to deal with their anxiety, and because they feel that male urge to 'do something'. Teaching men about their instinctive behaviours during birth and how to work with them is a much more empowering and constructive way of supporting BOTH father and mum. A father who is equipped with skills and understanding about birth and his role will be able to support mum in her wishes for her birth, give her oxytocin-boosting love and support, thus contributing even further to this aim of an empowered birth.

As an aside, I wonder whether some of these 'dad jokes' are actually an individual's way of trying to create a dialogue and rapport with the dad, or perhaps even indicate a nervousness in how to relate to the men and actually include them. Fathers themselves are well versed in this art of making a joke when they feel uncomfortable or uncertain – it is a natural way to cover up our nerves and unease! However, if we can support men to control this urge during birth, it is also important to support professionals to control it during their interactions with men. However, this first has to start with awareness of those behaviours and their impact, and a desire to want to become more father-inclusive, and an understanding and compassion for where men are coming from.

One paper (RCM, 2014) written to encourage father involvement highlighted the benefit of scheduling antenatal classes and appointments so as not to clash with football matches and suggested leaving 'male interest' magazines in the waiting room. If a father understands his presence is important, he will 'opt in' regardless of what is on TV or in the waiting room for him to read. Accessibility runs much deeper than this and it is at best a little insulting to assume that our gender naturally means we place football as a higher priority than our family. Treating partners with compassion, understanding and respect is the first step to really supporting a father to 'opt in' for the benefit for his family.

It is also worth considering how the names of the support/facilities can impact on the subconscious. If we want fathers to be involved and acknowledge how important they are, is this reflected and are they made to feel welcome, included and *important* when they are seeing events entitled: Breastfeeding Workshop for Mums (Dads welcome too). What about when they arrive at the 'Women and Baby Unit' – what is their place there? These messages take place usually on a more subconscious level, but this does not make the sense of displacement any less significant. If we make men feel from the outset that they are not really welcome, or are a 'visitor' or 'observer' then the subconscious often directs them to act accordingly, and thus we do a huge disservice to fathers, disempowering them at a time when their partner needs them to be empowered the most – to support her.

In the future, rather than 'midwife-led units', 'woman and baby units' or 'women-centred units' – I'd like to see just 'birth centres' or 'family-centred units' – neutral terminology which is truly centred on welcoming the birthing woman and whoever *she* has chosen to be her key supporters. In this way we are extending compassion and respect on a new level into the birthing arena.

Conclusion

And so I end where I began… empowerment of women in pregnancy and birth is long overdue. But consider this, if a woman's key supporter is the father of her child, what are you doing to *empower him*, so he in turn can *empower her* during the pregnancy, during the birth and for the rest of their lives as a family? Supporting fathers through education and respectful interactions will engage them more, and open up more

Recognising where we lack the knowledge or skill to be able to engage as compassionately and respectfully with fathers as we do with mothers is not a sign of weakness, but one of strength as it gives us the opportunity to address the imbalance.

It would be unthinkable for a professional to joke about how badly a woman was handling labour. It should not be acceptable to trivialize the feelings and experience of fathers and make similar 'jokes'. Fathers also deserve to be treated with compassion and respect, as they are vulnerable in their own way.

KEY MESSAGES

- Fathers have a crucial influence over the choices women are empowered to make in pregnancy, birth and early parenthood.
- Stereotyping fathers potentially sets up self-fulfilling prophecies and limits the potential of men as involved birth partners and fathers to the detriment of mum and baby.
- Increased awareness of our own interactions with men and how to make these more positive is crucial.
- Remember that the journey from a man to a dad is also one which is profound and full of emotions.

ACTION POINTS

- It's good to talk… and be quiet. Men are less verbal than women, in terms of their use of language and body language.
- Give dads information in a logical sequence as they are able to store it better for longer periods of time.
- Provide some space! Men tend to need more space than women when they are learning, due to the fact that they have lower serotonin levels and higher metabolism compared to women.
- Provide evidence. Men often enjoy understanding how something works – we are much more likely to be interested and remember it.
- Don't criticize us; it can affect our confidence levels, especially when it is about something we are already unsure of.
- Fathers also deserve to be treated with compassion and respect, as they are vulnerable in their own way.

8 Through the eyes of a doula

Kicki Hansard

In the years following the move of childbirth from the home to a hospital setting and in the shadow of the rise of obstetrics, some of the key components to facilitate physiological childbirth have fallen off our list of priorities. I'm feeling hopeful that we are waking up and opening our eyes to see how the culture of maternity services is heading in the wrong direction. So when I was invited to contribute to this book, as a mother and a doula, I knew exactly what I would like to share with you.

Mothering the mother

When I hear the words kindness, compassion and respect, people like Mother Teresa, Mahatma Gandhi and Nelson Mandela spring to my mind. All of them seemed to encompass these human qualities in abundance and became well known for displaying an array of ways to express to others these gifts that they were born with. However, I would like to suggest another person that we are all familiar with, who is amongst us and often is working the magic of compassion and kindness in the background of every family – the mother!

I don't think it was a coincidence that mothering the mother was the phrase used by Klaus, Kennell and Klaus (1993) when they wrote the book with the same name about doulas and the support that doulas provide. A doula is a person, usually a woman, who provides emotional, practical and informative support to women and their families before, during and after childbirth. Just like a doula needs to be adaptable, resourceful and often creative to meet all the different needs of the mother and family that she is supporting, a mother needs the exact same qualities when supporting each of her children, her partner and the extended family.

Listening and hearing!

I believe that if we were to view every person we come across, as we care for women and their families, as our children, who might be feeling fearful and apprehensive about what may lie ahead of them, we might be able to connect in a more empathetic way. Seeing that there is a need that is not being met, a fear of something, we can approach them like we would approach a child who is scared of the 'monster under the bed' or has a stomach ache and doesn't want to go to school. If we think as a mother, we know that we need to take a little more time to listen to what our child is saying, to join

53

in the dance of exploring in a non-judgemental way to find out how to support them as best as possible during what to them is a difficult time. We can't dismiss or minimize the issues and make it unimportant as this is something that requires compassion and patience. We might feel that what we are faced with is going to take up a lot of our time and cause us a delay, which will mess up the rest of our day. However, if we can see in this woman what we can see in our own child, someone who needs us to give them some of our time to really hear them, we can generously give them this precious gift – the gift of time. The very fact that doulas exists and are a growing profession (with a small p) shows that these special mothering qualities are missing from maternity services at the moment, an ancient custom which still exists in tribal communities.

It's easy to put blame and judgement on the person who is 'making us feel' a certain way instead of identifying what the need is in us that is not being met. We all have the choice to react to events and people around us in either a compassionate or judgemental way. If in our heads we might be thinking *what's her problem, I'm only trying to help* or *does she not think I know what I'm doing?* when faced with a woman who is questioning guidelines for example, and wanting time to speak to her husband or perhaps doula before 'allowing' straightforward procedures which might take place in the hospital. However, if we do, we are making an assumption about her behaviour, or judgements as to why she is making our job so difficult. Instead, we could choose to connect with this woman, to try and discover what her needs are and what we can do to meet those needs. Perhaps we might engage in a conversation where we listen compassionately by hearing what she is fearful of and also explaining to her what the needs are for us as the care provider. The usual response from someone who hears criticism or judgements is to invest all their energy into a counterattack or jump into self-defence.

As a mother, we might sometimes find ourselves in a situation where our child needs empathy and we assume that he/she wants reassurance or advice on how to fix a problem and our child ends up feeling frustrated and unsupported. As this is the perceived role of an expert or medical professional, it can be even more of a challenge to change the belief that every situation needs to be fixed or some advice needs to be handed out. However, this intellectual way of approaching a challenge will usually block the person from being totally present with what is being communicated and makes empathy difficult. If we want to communicate in a compassionate way, we need to look beyond the words that people might be using when expressing themselves and really listen for their feelings, needs and requests.

What makes women choose?

During my 12 years as a doula, I have worked with survivors of sexual abuse, recovering drug-addicts, same-sex couples, women with anxiety disorders and other mental health issues and women and partners traumatized by previous birth experiences. What I have found is that by connecting to them in an empathetic way, I am learning to hear their needs and feelings. It is not always obvious from the outset as one of my clients told me in our antenatal meeting that she wanted to have an epidural as soon as she was in labour. I'm a big believer in supporting women's choices but I also like to hear, if they are willing to share, their reasons behind their choice so I can fully understand where they are coming from and authentically support them. I said to her: '*It sounds like you have pretty strong feelings about having an epidural, would you be willing to share with me why?*' Her answer did surprise me a bit as she said: '*I just want to make sure that if I need stitches, I will not be able to feel them.*' So, this woman was not worried about labour or contractions but it was afterwards, just in case she needed to have some repair work done, that she wanted to be numb. I have learnt to never assume why someone is making a specific request or is behaving in a certain way because I know that I would most likely be wrong in my judgement.

I have also witnessed some wonderful demonstrations of kindness and respect from maternity workers, totally committed to woman-centred care and understanding of the impact a birth experience can have on a woman. I can recall a time when an obstetrician warmed the forceps in warm water to make it more comfortable for the mum and the baby, and he told her what a wonderful job she had done and how he was simply going to support her in the very last little bit of pushing her baby out. The parents, despite the many unwanted interventions, could not stop talking about what a great birth it had been. Another time, the midwife discussed the reasons with the obstetrician why he should avoid performing an episiotomy during a vacuum extraction. The woman was too exhausted to speak up for herself but the midwife had read the birth preferences and could tell how important it was for this woman not to be cut; the baby was born without any damage to the perineum.

Communication is a main tool in the toolbox of a doula and I would encourage more of this kind of training for all maternity professionals. Some more emphasis put on personal development and interpersonal skills would be of great benefit. Doula courses focus on getting the doula to start reflecting on her behaviour, to recognize her own triggers and be aware of what language she uses with her clients and the maternity professionals she will be working alongside. I believe that by creating community and working together within our different roles, remembering that the focus should always be on the woman and her family, and that each and every woman and family we work with have their unique set of needs and requirements, we will be able to make huge improvements in women's experiences of birth.

Conclusion

A doula's aim is to work with her head, heart and 'gut feeling' in equal measures – too much in her head and she will fall into the system that traps midwives and doctors, worrying about what *could* happen – too much with her heart and she will be rescuing women which leads to disempowering rather than empowerment and, last but not least, intuition, which is something that develops and grows over time. I am learning that, by using my mothering skills, the more I can connect to everyone with kindness, compassion and respect and I have become better at listening to what my gut is telling me at times when I am at a loss, both as a doula and as a mother – the two roles magically intertwine.

KEY MESSAGES

- Empathy is the respectful perception of what others are experiencing and we need to connect caringly to the women we look after to be able to show empathy.
- Ensure that you are speaking a language that is non-judgemental and doesn't limit choices.
- Instead of there being 'them' and 'us', let's create a community where we all show kindness, compassion and respect to each other, ourselves and our clients.

ACTION POINTS

- Become an explorer with the women you meet and care for – look at them with the eyes of a mother to connect compassionately.
- Stay present and focus on what is going on right now in this moment – be generous and give them the gift of time.
- Take ownership of your own feelings and needs – you have a choice to react judgementally or compassionately to the events and people around you.
- Be respectful of the choices women make – discover what their needs are so you can fulfil that need yourself or refer to someone that can.
- There is always a reason for the way we all behave – identify those reasons in the women you support and in yourself – show kindness to both.

9 Promoting normal birth: courage through compassion

Tracey Cooper

I believe in a woman's infinite ability to give birth to her baby. I consider myself a protector of this ability from interference, unless it will improve the outcome. Whilst supporting women to give birth I believe care should be centred around the woman, and delivered with compassion.

Compassionate care helps the woman to cope with the birth process, and facilitates her ability to birth her baby as naturally as possible. Compassion is linked to courage. If we are challenged in our ability to provide compassionate care to women, we need courage to speak up and to initiate or support change.

This chapter presents my personal story of trying to remain true to compassionate care in practice. I empathize strongly with midwives, and with others providing maternity care, who continually struggle to provide woman-centred compassionate care, and to support normal physiological birth processes. My intention in this chapter is to try to encourage care-givers in this area to keep on, and to value what they are doing. It's like a chain; if one person can help others by demonstrating compassionate care as much as possible, then others can take courage from this and provide a role model in their turn. This way, we can all work together to make it happen for all women, babies, and families.

The importance of compassionate woman-centred care

'*Compassion is the* emotion *that one feels in response to the suffering of others that motivates a desire to help.*' Oxford English Dictionary, 2000

Conceptually, compassion can be seen as the response that is generated by a feeling of empathic distress, which is characterized by the feeling of distress in relation to another person's suffering (Goetz *et al*, 2010; Hoffman, 1981, Ekman, 2003). This perspective of compassion is based on the observation that people sometimes feel and even emulate the emotions of those around them (Hatfield, 1993).

In terms of childbirth, this might be less about women suffering per se, and more about their need for support to prevent distress and suffering from occurring. In this respect, compassion could be said to be like the growth of a tree. It has to develop strong roots within care giving. It needs to push up above the soil into the sunlight, to make a real difference, and it has to grow strong like the tree trunk, upwards through organizations and society as a whole. The leaves and branches have to infiltrate outwards, to positively influence perceptions of childbirth, and to then, in turn, encourage compassionate care that respects physiology and to reduce the fear that has become engrained into current maternity services.

Getting there: my story

Personally, I gained the desire to make a difference to women's birth experiences through listening to women and understanding why compassionate care was important to them. As a student midwife and later as a junior midwife, working alongside different mentors influenced my practice. I worked with some exceptional role models who positively influenced how I cared for women; conversely I worked with others who made me determined never to emulate any part of their practice.

When I was a student midwife my community midwife mentor had the highest home birth rate and supported the local birth centre. She also was a perfect example of providing true compassionate care to women. I spent most of my community experience with her, and she had a huge influence on my practice. She taught me how to commit to women through compassion, and how to make it the best experience possible for them.

Learning to be courageous

Later on I worked as the manager of an alongside birth centre, and I used the skills learnt from the mentor mentioned above. It was during this time that I was able to demonstrate how compassionate woman-centred care made a difference to women's experiences. Being an advocate for women and midwives was to become the bedrock of my practice. This is where I learnt to be brave and to stand up for woman-centred compassionate care.

Following a few meetings with key leaders in the organization, in relation to the local birth centre, I realized that this precious place was to be obliterated. This was bad news indeed. Even though the birth centre was small, the outcomes for mothers and babies, and the mothers' experiences of birth, were excellent. Midwives loved working in this environment. If there was any hope that the birth centre had a future, someone needed to act quickly. It didn't take long for me to realize that this person had to be me. I had as a mantra the line 'You've only got three choices in life: give up; give in; or give it all you've got'.

Several difficult meetings took place and I persisted in making the case to keep the birth centre open. I used the evidence and women's voices of their experiences to make the birth centre bigger to accommodate more women. The team hadn't expected that! Indeed, the birth centre wasn't closed, it was developed, and we received an award from the Royal College of Midwives in 2002 for working in partnership with women and for midwifery innovation.

Being courageous together

In a different maternity service in another region in England, I met an amazingly strong group of midwives who were distressed by the closure of their freestanding birth centre. I worked with them to try to reopen the centre. When this failed, I personally felt I had let them down, but there was no support for us to achieve it at the highest level of the organization.

I then worked with them to channel their energies into another avenue. They reinvigorated themselves to continue their passion and commitment to promoting home birth instead, doubling their previous home birth rates. The midwives felt that they could use their skills in promoting normal birth to achieve not only greater satisfaction for women, but for their own professional satisfaction. Their passion for the job they were doing was interpreted as the 'food of their soul'. They won 'Team of the Year' at the *British Journal of Midwifery* Awards in 2008 and I am and always will be very proud of them turning a bad situation into something good.

Feeling disempowered and insignificant can lead to despair, and be a barrier to providing compassionate care. I worked with midwives in another organization who felt that the midwifery leadership was generating an oppressive culture. I listened to them and collated their stories along with Sarah, an extraordinary midwife, who demonstrated enormous courage through being willing to speak up and address this issue too. Many other midwives then gained courage and shared their stories. We all stood together to try to improve the culture for the sake of women using the service, and for each other. The Supervisors of Midwives (SOMs) were incredibly supportive to the midwives through this difficult time and were instrumental in making this change happen. They were given support from the Local Supervising Authority Midwifery Officer (The LSAMO puts the responsibilities of the LSA into practice and this work cannot be delegated to another person or another role. The LSAMO is a practising midwife who provides leadership, support and guidance primarily on midwifery practice and the supervision of midwives.) We all worked together to make the change happen. This period of time was very difficult for all of us, but if we hadn't acted when we did, nothing would have changed.

In particular, Sarah and I knew we were stepping outside usual boundaries; we were standing out and being so-called 'tall poppies' by taking the issue forward. Indeed, we felt very much that we were likely to have our heads chopped off with the gardening shears! But, as my previous experiences had taught me, if we don't act when difficult situations arise that we believe to be wrong, nothing will change. If the midwives had not had the courage to help take this forward, we knew that the oppressive culture that prevailed at the time would not have changed.

Following this period the culture improved, becoming progressive, forward thinking, and more compassionate, both for women and for staff.

Success breeds success. In the same area discussed above, a freestanding birth centre that was in danger of closing due to low usage was saved, and it is now thriving. Because of the success of this venture and the evidence available, investment was made to develop another alongside birth centre. I believe this happened as a result of engaging the hearts and minds of all involved. Having the courage to support the kind of maternity care settings that encourage relationship-based care is crucial. In my own research, for example, I found that women who received a midwifery-led model of care felt empowered to deal with the normal birth process by their midwife (Cooper and Lavender, 2013).

Through a local midwives network I met Susan, a supervisor of midwives, who informed me about a practice issue, which was affecting the care of women, potentially negatively influencing outcomes for mothers and babies. I supported her by providing her with evidence that the intervention was inappropriate and potentially harmful to present to senior managers, resulting in a temporary withdrawal of the treatment. Unfortunately the decision was reversed again, and once more all women experiencing an uncomplicated pregnancy were encouraged to have electronic fetal monitoring. I provided assistance to Susan throughout this period, so that she was enabled to support her midwifery colleagues and the women they were caring for. I needed to encourage Susan as the situation felt hopeless; there appeared to be an overriding belief from some of the leading clinicians and managers that medical intervention was the only solution to a particular problem, and a failure to acknowledge potential harm.

Even though I wasn't employed there, I was invited to a meeting to discuss the issue. My argument was that they were not providing compassionate care, as they were not giving evidence-based care, and that there was potential for harm with the use of the intervention. I highlighted current evidence, and together with midwives and obstetricians tried to influence the decision. This was to no avail, the recommendation for the intervention continued. I lobbied for change in the background, liaising with professional organisations and colleagues. These actions resulted in the advice to all mothers to have the intervention being withdrawn. Susan was courageous, brave enough to speak out when she knew something was wrong. I tried to support her, and act as a catalyst for change. I couldn't accept that women were being subjected to unnecessary medicalisation and at best potentially disrupting the natural rhythms of labour and birth, at worst possibly causing harm (NICE 2014). I also felt compelled to help midwives who were distressed by the actions. When maternity care workers collaborate during times of stress or uncertainty, they can maximise potential to make a difference.

Influencing the national maternity agenda

It is possible to bring beliefs about the need for compassionate maternity care into the national as well as the local arena. For example, I have recently been a member of a national clinical guideline development group, related to intrapartum care (NICE, 2014). My desire to be involved in the project stemmed from believing in women's ability to give birth physiologically in most cases. I also believe that compassionate care is a fundamental element of enabling a positive birth experience, and that compassion and courage are inextricably linked. I upheld this philosophy throughout the meetings and related work, and even though there were times when it was difficult when members of the group didn't agree. We all worked incredibly hard and we did reach consensus on everything eventually, but on some days I cried with frustration. On the other hand, there were moments when I felt euphoric because conclusions drawn from the evidence felt groundbreaking and had the potential to make a huge difference to childbearing women, maternity care workers and maternity services in general. I had to make sure I made every opportunity count by inputting wisely and compassionately into the development of this clinical guidance. Now it's up to those using it to decide what impact it will have (NICE, 2014).

Conclusion

From feeling compassion for women during birth through to using it to influence others at local, regional, and national levels, we all can do it. If we work with each other to make a difference we can move mountains. As a final note I would like to pay tribute and offer my gratitude to the academics and researchers who have provided the evidence base for caring and compassionate maternity services – the fuel for the passion that stimulates practitioners and others to make the necessary changes to support woman-centred compassionate maternity care design and provision.

KEY MESSAGES

- If we are challenged in our ability to provide compassionate care to women, we need courage to speak up and to initiate or support change.
- When maternity care workers collaborate during times of stress or uncertainty, they can maximize potential to make a difference.

ACTION POINTS

- Don't sit and watch when you feel something is wrong: do something about it. Stand up for what you believe in, if you can.
- Use available evidence to influence change. If you don't know whether research is available, ask for help via your colleagues, local university, or via social media.
- Be brave – yes, it's scary, but if you don't try it you will never know that you can!
- Work together – we are stronger in numbers.
- YOU CAN make a difference. '*Success is not final, failure is not fatal: it is the courage to continue that counts.*' – Winston Churchill

10 Not all obstetricians

My chapter is about a bad day at work. This day was not the worst day at work I've ever had. It was just an ordinary, difficult day that followed an ordinary, difficult night on call. I've had other such bad days, and they often slam up against my life outside of medicine. You probably have had them too. Post call, on your way home exhausted after the stress of doing an inadequate job with inadequate pay and inadequate resources and inadequate rest, you are berated by a grocery store cashier for having thirteen items in the twelve-items-or-less line. Reflexes slowed by fatigue, you didn't notice the light changed to green fast enough, the person in the car behind you leans on their horn and shoots you the finger. You can see their face contorted in a snarl as they squeal past you. You cry, but it's not just about the driver. It's about all of it: it's about your own inadequacy, the inadequacy of the system, about how human beings can be so mean.

My chapter is also from a little blog I write. It only has a few posts, and I'm certainly not advertising that you drop everything and read it. I post things only periodically, irregularly, when I have time, which is not very often. I started the blog when I read another blog, written by midwife Sheena Byrom, about how to fix the broken maternity system. It made me think about how bad maternity systems happen to good people.

Lastly, my chapter is about a bad day in the patriarchy. As if there are any other kinds of days. From my point of view, there's no point in denying it: the field of obstetrics was mostly planted by men. As I see it, misogyny and the abuse of women were mixed up in it at the start. We can't ignore that history, and if we are to dig up the system and replant it with kindness and compassion, we must search for and pull up the roots of paternalistic medicine.

* * *

In Tolkien's classic *The Lord of the Rings*, Arwen Evenstar gives up her immortality for the love of a mortal man, Aragorn. Arwen's father is against the match. He's got nothing against Aragorn, it's just that he understands the full weight of her choice. But Arwen won't be dissuaded. We often do things that are crazy in the state of temporary insanity induced by love. Like having children. It'd make a great story if I could say that's why I did obstetrics too. For the love of it. But looking back, it might have been for hate.

My son Colin, the philosopher, tells me that our decisions go back to the big bang if we go back far enough. By this he means that there's a certain inevitability to our choices. That if we look backwards at our lives, everything that happens nudges us in a certain direction, and we find ourselves falling down a particular pathway under the influence of these unseen forces. That hateful obstetrician whom I met the day I attended my first ever birth might have tripped me up a little, but I might have been heading in that direction too.

I like to think that the reason I became an obstetrician was that when I saw that doctor pull that baby out with forceps for no apparent reason, it made me think that I could do better. That I could cancel out some of the abuses that I saw were happening to women. The trouble is that some of those things I did to cancel out the wrongs have been acts of responsible subversion. Because they maintain the status quo, responsible subversion is somewhat irresponsible. And also, since people don't know about my good deeds, one day history might judge me in the same light as those evil obstetricians. History might think I was one of them. But history lies sometimes. Like, just because I once owned a gold lamé pantsuit, it doesn't mean I was a disco queen. Disco music gave me a migraine in my ear.

I've written about Mary Rose McCall's book *The Birth Wars* before. In it, she compares the philosophical disagreements between midwives and obstetricians (birth as natural: birth as dangerous) to a war in which women and babies are the collateral damage. I'm aware that one day my grandchildren might well ask me what side of the war I was on. If you read the obstetric history books it would appear that all my predecessors were monsters and maybe they were but more likely they were just human beings trying to do the best they could with the material they had to work with: the lowest human life forms on the planet – mothers and babies. Who knows, maybe Joseph Delee himself, he of forceps = gentle / vagina = skull-crusher fame, may have been a closet feminist.

The poet and philosopher Criss Jami wrote '*When good people consider you the bad guy, you develop a heart to help the bad ones. You try to understand them.*' And he's right. In trying to understand the field of obstetrics we must consider the patriarchy, and the fact that birth must not go quietly into the service of those dark knights.

In the world of obstetrics, there are too many bad guys. Not all obstetricians, that's for sure, but far too many. The sad explanation is that we do not value motherhood, which is a nice way of saying that our culture (still) hates women. I know many people won't believe that: they will say they love women, but they only love good women, thin women, beautiful young women, they don't love women on welfare, women who smoke and who eat junk food, women with rotten teeth and rolls of fat, women who have had too many babies by too many different men.

When I had my first baby one of the first things I felt was a deep connection to all of the other women who had babies before me. This feeling surprised me. I think part of the reason it surprised me was, in truth, that I had been a snob. Before I became a mother myself I hadn't appreciated the profundity of the act. After all, even stupid women become mothers. Women with rotten teeth, and rolls of fat, who eat too much junk food. These women are often, too often, some might say, mothers too. If ordinary, regular women could do this thing – become mothers – like I just had, then perhaps there was more to them then met the eye. Maybe there were other things I'd overlooked. It wouldn't be the first time I'd judged someone harshly and then come to find things out about them that shattered my image not only of them but also of myself as a fair minded and reasonable person. What all women have in common is that when they become mothers they deserve the best of care. Let that sink in. That woman with the tattoos and badly dyed hair who got addicted and had a baby with a gang member deserves the best of care. Yes, we have a duty to protect the baby from abuse from her own flawed mother. But the best way of doing that is to make the world a better place so that good mothering can emerge from flawed women.

The Lord of the Rings trilogy has a long appendix, so maybe you haven't read it. In it we find out what happens to Arwen in the end. As it gets closer to that day of reckoning, when Aragorn ages and eventually dies, Arwen comes to regret her decision. The reality of a mortal life is before her. It is in the end, looking back, where choices can be regretted. When we suffer, ourselves, for taking what stances we took in our lives. Where what seems like a good idea at the time doesn't seem like such a great idea after all. Part of this is just what always happens when we have lived a while in the actual life we chose, with all of its disappointments. The road we didn't take often seems so much better, because it's always a fantasy. We don't imagine alternative careers to be boring, alternative spouses to be abusive, alternative children that won't brush their teeth when asked.

Imagine Arwen sitting at the coffee table with her best friend. There are things even best friends don't talk about, for example, their choice of partner, especially when it's a done deal like that. My dearest friends have ended up with some surprising choices. I know left wing beauties married to right wing uglies; down-to-earth earth mothers hitched to conservative snobs; friends who divorced weirdos and remarried idiots. You can't account for it other than thinking that Cupid is pretty random.

We might not comment but we certainly think it: what the hell did she see in him and she could have done so much better. Behind her back Arwen's friends might have said that Aragorn was pretty hot in the day and a King and all, but seriously, I'm sure she coulda had any pick of the elves *and* kept her immortality. To paraphrase my grandmother, it's just as easy to marry a mortal man as it is to marry an immortal one.

We tell ourselves it's for a just and worthy cause, this diminishment of power. But there is no reward for love in the patriarchy. Most women become lesser beings there, in the service of men. We tell ourselves it's okay, we've done it for a noble cause: because we love them. And we are punished, because they – the ones that write the rules that govern how women are abused and oppressed – they hate us most of all.

* * *

I am leaving the hospital after a difficult night which stretched well into the next day. A colleague has called in sick, and I have stayed far beyond the end of my shift. When I get to my car, I realize that in my haste to arrive in a crushing emergency, I have parked in the space reserved for the paediatrician on call. My driver's side window is plastered with a sticker warning me that I will be towed if this transgression ever happens again. The sticker obstructs my vision and I can't remove it. I cheer myself up by indulging in a fantasy about what happens if I am killed in a car accident on my way home. The CEO of the hospital attends my funeral, the jerk who is a member of the hospital board, and wait, here is a particular manager who has previously made my life miserable; they all say how great I was. It makes at least page three of the *Times*. The dream sequence fades into nightmare when a man approaches. I think he's going to offer me sympathy for a moment; he is looking at the sticker, so I get a shock, because he's nasty. He strides towards me menacingly. How dare I park in this spot, he (An Important Man!) had An Important Meeting!! in the morning and was Running Late!!! I try to explain about the emergency c section that turned into a postpartum haemorrhage and the fetal distress that followed in the room next door, and at the same time and to top it off there was a woman with an intrauterine death who I have just left and how one thing led to the other and that I didn't mean it, I try to engender some sympathy, you see, while I appreciate the importance of the meeting, there were lives truly at stake, except for that woman with the dead baby which wasn't a physical emergency but it was an emotional one, when I realize he doesn't care. All I manage to say, hanging my head, is that I was on call. He knows what it's like to be on call, he's done it himself for years, as he (raising his voice) – don't I know – is a Consultant Paediatrician. It doesn't dawn on me until later when I am at home, that, because of my crappy car, and my crappy clothes, and maybe the mascara tracks on my face from the dead baby, he treats me that way because he doesn't see me as a peer.

He thinks I am a midwife.

KEY MESSAGES

- Doctors are privileged members of the medical team, high up the chain of command, and by definition this privilege means we are sheltered from the difficulties our midwifery and nursing colleagues face on a day to day basis.
- Women must not be the victims in the professional battles of maternity care workers.
- Obstetrics involves many women as 'patients', and the workforce. Our patriarchal society doesn't value motherhood enough, and it doesn't value women's work. Understanding this point is key to building compassion and, ultimately, positive change in all aspects of the work.
- Not all obstetricians are insensitive, unkind, or uncaring practitioners, although they may not see the privileged place they inhabit within the maternity system.

ACTION POINTS

- A hard day at work doesn't always stay there. If you have one, tell someone about it, or write it down.
- Try to look at the world from the point of view of others in the maternity system. The obstetric voice is not the only voice that matters.
- Work at seeing all others as deserving of compassion and kindness, and all members of your team equally deserving of respect.
- When others let you down, extend compassion.

11 We can learn to be caring

Robin Youngson

Qualities such as empathy, kindness and compassion are often perceived to be inborn personality traits – some practitioners have them and others don't. Recent scandals in the National Health Service (NHS) and beyond have highlighted a lack of compassion in patient care and one of the responses is to propose values-based recruitment, with the presumption that compassion is an innate quality that can be identified and selected. Other authorities call for compassion to be included in the curriculum for the training of health professionals but there are real questions about the possibility of teaching compassion.

However, compassion is a complex construct, including elements of empathy, sympathy, sensitivity, non-judgement, tolerance of distress, and motivation. Recent research suggests that some of the elements can be enhanced with formal training. But maybe life experience is a better teacher? Some say that compassion can be 'caught' rather than 'taught'.

What is certain is that the performance of health professionals in aspects of kindness, caring, empathy and compassion can develop over time. Given that compassion is a motivation to respond to suffering – more than just a feeling or emotion – personal attitude plays a major role. Attitudes can change. This is the story of my long journey from detached clinical to compassionate practitioner and the insights I gained along the way.

A lack of physician empathy can lead to emotional trauma for the patient

The patient was having an emergency caesarean section under epidural anaesthesia. She was extremely anxious, exhausted and tearful. When the surgeon made a move, the patient yelped. 'I can feel it!' she said.

Her husband was staring at me, wild-eyed! 'Do something!' he implored.

I was the on-call anaesthesia resident. Caring for patients having emergency caesarean section was a stressful event. As trainees, we were taught how dangerous was a general anaesthetic: it affected the baby as well as the mother, there was risk of stomach contents regurgitating into the lungs, and tracheal intubation was often difficult in the pregnant patient. Failed intubation could lead to death.

Epidural anaesthesia was a safer option for both mother and baby but the surgery was often a difficult ordeal for the patient. Even with the best anaesthetic, the exhausted and frightened mother had to put up with many discomforts. But epidural anaesthesia was not all that reliable – too often the patient experienced discomfort or even pain.

I was stressed and sweating. I tried my best to reassure the patient. I offered and gave doses of painkiller, and even gas to breathe. The patient continued to cry out. Her husband was at the bedside in the operating theatre, obviously distressed. He started to get angry.

'Why isn't the anaesthesia working? Do you know what you are doing?!'

I did my best to reassure and placate him. I was extremely reluctant to administer full general anaesthesia, half-way through surgery. Somehow we got through to the end of the operation.

The husband was furious: 'Why did you let her suffer so much pain?'

To my shame I responded, 'Well, that's much less pain than she would have had during normal childbirth.'

Talk about lack of empathy!

It's the only time in my career that I've faced a formal patient complaint. I endured two painful and humiliating interviews with this angry family. I felt ashamed at my lack of empathy and bitterly regretted the throw-away remark I had made under the stress of the situation.

I started life as an engineer, then became a doctor. I revelled in the technical aspects of medicine, and especially anaesthetic practice. But at the time I was lacking the skills of compassionate caring and unaware how much my detached attitude could harm patients.

Now I'm the co-founder of an international movement for compassionate, human-centred healthcare. What changed? How did I learn to be more compassionate?

Choosing to love your job

My greatest teacher proved to be an unforgettable patient. Jessie was 85 years old, had bowel cancer, and barely survived each day owing to a life-threatening heart condition. I had the unenviable job of anaesthetising her for major surgery.

She attended the hospital in a wheelchair, looking crumpled and lopsided owing to a devastating stroke she'd suffered twenty years before. Her left side was paralyzed. She was overweight and the tissues of her face sagged in untidy folds like an unmade bed. Jessie had only half a smile but there was mischief and light in her eyes. She still managed to live alone and I quickly began to sense an indomitable spirit.

Jessie was in big trouble. Her bowel cancer was bleeding and she was very anaemic. The tumour was partly obstructing her bowel and it was hard for her to eat. The colicky abdominal pains were troublesome.

In addition to her devastating stroke, Jessie had many other medical risk factors. Her aortic heart valve was calcified and severely narrowed. Her coronary arteries were clogged. She teetered on the edge of a heart attack and suffered frequent attacks of chest pain.

I concluded that Jessie had only a fifty per cent chance of surviving her operation and that her prospects of ever leaving hospital were dismal.

With a heavy heart, I did my best to explain to Jessie the enormity of the surgical risk.

In a surprising gesture, she took my hand in hers. 'Robin, I put my faith in you. I know you'll do the best job you can and God will be watching over you.'

I struggled to maintain what I thought then was the proper clinical detachment. I felt embarrassed and was anxious for this uncomfortable consultation to end.

On the eve of surgery I felt duty bound to explain again the dire risks she was facing. Jessie interrupted my listing of the perils. 'Robin, you're looking so worried about giving my anaesthetic that I think I need to cheer you up. I'm going to tell you a joke!'

Lifting her forefinger up to touch her lips, she blew a lopsided and wet-sounding raspberry. 'What's that?' she said!

'I have no idea,' I replied, shaking my head in confusion.

'It's a fart trying to get past a g-string!' she exclaimed with a wicked twinkle in her eye.

Jessie had a stormy time in surgery and post-operative care. She narrowly scraped through several crises, never once complaining. I went to see her again, three days after surgery.

She held my hand again. 'Robin, I prayed that you would survive my anaesthetic, and you did!'

Jessie, with devastating effectiveness, undid all of my clinical defences and gave me an experience of shared humanity. She used one of the most powerful tools at our disposal – humour and laughter. It was the start of my journey of personal healing. It's something I try to teach my colleagues, the stepping aside from professional and expert roles to simply be a caring human being.

But Jessie's most important lesson was about choosing an attitude.

She wasn't grumpy or ill tempered. She didn't complain. She didn't dwell on her misfortune. She chose instead to show concern and compassion for me as a vulnerable human being. She gave me support, she cheered me up, and she told me a joke!

If Jessie could choose humour, laughter and compassion in her awful circumstances, then what excuse do we health professionals have to be grumpy or feel sorry for ourselves?

Many years later, the thought came to me at 4am while driving to the hospital to attend a woman in childbirth. I was the on-call anaesthetist, summoned to perform an epidural injection for pain relief.

I was exhausted, bad-tempered, resentful and feeling sorry for myself. After a busy day this was my fourth call of the night. I had been in bed only ten minutes after the last call-out and I was angry that the midwife hadn't contacted me when I was already in the hospital.

I tended to carry my resentment into work with me and was sometimes intolerant of frustrations, delays or missing equipment. It wasn't always the friendliest of receptions when I entered the labour room. Sometimes it felt like I was the enemy, the 'wicked' doctor interfering in the natural process of childbirth when the Birth Plan certainly didn't include medical interventions!

Finding the right equipment, gaining the midwife's help in positioning the patient for the epidural injection, and communicating instructions, felt like an uphill struggle. Sometimes the epidural didn't work well and I'd be called out of bed again.

As I drove into the hospital with all these negative thoughts and feelings, I suddenly felt ashamed. Jessie's spirit came to me. What right did I have to feel grumpy and sorry for myself when I was being invited to take part in an intimate and life-changing event?

I decided at that moment that every time I was called out I would dispel negative thoughts and instead reflect on the extraordinary privilege of what I was called to do: relieve pain and transform the experience for a vulnerable patient.

So now I take great care with the spirit and presence I bring to the patient. I enter the labour room softly with compassion and gentleness. I notice how this affects the mother in reducing fear and distress.

I greet and acknowledge the other people in the room. I ask the midwife if she has been busy and when she last had any sleep or rest. I do the epidural injection with the minimum of fuss and then witness the miracle of pain relief. It is a joyous experience. I don't care how tired I am. I go home with love and joy in my heart.

How amazingly the world changed when I chose to have a different attitude!

Sometimes I thought the midwives resented my coming to do an epidural. Some were surly and uncommunicative, they would neglect to introduce me to the patient or other family members in the room, I would have to ask for assistance, the equipment wouldn't be ready.

Now I feel like an honoured visitor. I am greeted warmly. I have the sense that my praises have been sung to the patient even before I step into the labour room. The midwife thoughtfully prepares for my arrival, finding all the equipment and positioning the patient ready for the procedure. I find that the pain relief is more effective and the rate of complications is greatly reduced.

It's as if all the grumpy and difficult midwives have had a personality transplant – and they probably thought the same about me!

For most of my career, I considered the problem of the relationship with midwives as an external problem, a consequence of their difficult attitude and behaviour. My more recent experience leads me to believe that the problem, and certainly the solution, existed in my own head. The only person who changed was 'me' but the consequence of that was a remarkable change in my whole world experience.

Sometimes you have to change 'me' to change the world.

As my practice deepened I began to reflect on my professional role, how I might best serve my patients and where I might find the deepest joy and satisfaction. I came to realize that for much of my career, my identity and self-esteem were wrapped up in being a highly trained technical expert.

I was always friendly and helpful but I was certainly the person in charge of the agenda. If my patients had questions beyond the scope of my technical expertise, I was skilled at diverting them back onto safer ground.

Over time, I have gradually re-conceptualized my role as that of a caring human being first and an expert second. That enabled me to be more humble and respectful, to listen patiently, to form more trusting relationships with my patients and to bring much greater compassion and humanity to the relationship.

I began to take great pleasure in helping patients in whatever way I could, regardless of whether or not it related to my specific technical role as an anaesthetist. After all, the complexity of healthcare is bewildering for patients and we have many opportunities to help them navigate the system and find the help they need.

I've come to realize that the most powerful way to improve your work experience, and to enhance your wellbeing, happiness and resilience is to CHOOSE TO LOVE YOUR WORK.

Make a deliberate choice about where you focus your attention. Every single day, healthcare offers opportunities for deep pleasure, satisfaction and meaning in the connection with patients and families. Take pleasure in the smallest things. Be mindful of the attitude you bring to each patient encounter.

The latest research from the growing field of positive psychology shows that gratitude and appreciation are two of the most important practices for enhancing positivity, happiness and wellbeing (Fredrickson, 2010). Appreciation is a habit to be developed, not an inborn personality trait.

Expressing appreciation to others strongly enhances social bonds. When you bring this attitude to your care of patients, you will find that patients respond much more positively, you'll enjoy your work more, and suffer fewer complaints. Teamwork will be enhanced.

So we come back to the patient from my story at the beginning of the chapter. She's pregnant again and booked for an elective caesarean.

How do I, as the anaesthetist, care for a patient like this who has been deeply traumatized by the experience of a 'nightmare' caesarean? With my new-found knowledge, attitude and skills, it's now become one of the most gratifying tasks I ever do in medicine: helping a patient heal past trauma and create a joyful experience in childbirth.

Here's what I do.

The first greeting is important. I take care with the spirit I bring into the room. I knock on the door and ask permission to enter. I introduce myself to the patient and her partner. I don't just give my title but I explain my role and intention. 'My job is to administer the anaesthetic and make sure you feel comfortable and safe. I want this to be a joyous experience for you.'

I ask permission to sit on the patient's bed and wait for the 'OK'. Every action I take is carefully calibrated to give the patient a sense of control.

When we're done with introduction and I'm settled comfortably at the patient's level, I ask, 'How are you?'

I love this moment. I sit with all senses wide open to witness the response. Almost all patients display some anxiety. I might remark, "You're looking a bit apprehensive – did you get any sleep last night?" And I validate their feelings, 'It's natural to feel apprehensive, it just proves you're a human being like everyone else.' I smile and wait for their response.

My empathy often elicits further signs of fear. I ask if the patient is just a bit nervous or if there is any particular issue causing concern? I enquire about the thoughts that were going around the patient's head at 3am when lying awake.

This often uncovers the story of the previous trauma. I take care to empathize with the patient and to show how seriously I take her experience. I don't make any excuses or try to defend the medical practice – after all, the end result for the patient was severe distress. I will attempt to interpret what happened from a medical point of view so that we can avoid the same problems today. If I have the medical charts, I'll examine them together with the patient. I'll explain what I'm looking for, what I have found, and how we can interpret the findings in the light of the patient's story.

One patient told me a horrifying story about anaesthetic side-effects. She was overdosed with the spinal anaesthetic. As a consequence, her blood pressure dropped dangerously. Her husband said she went 'white as a sheet', became agitated, and started vomiting. The patient told me she thought she was going to die. At that point the anaesthetist decided that things were getting out of control so he sent the husband out of the operating room. The only person available to take him away was the patient's trusted midwife. At the moment the patient thought she was going to die, the two people who most cared for her were removed from the room. She felt utterly alone. When she told me this story, it was evident she was deeply traumatized by these events. She'd had nightmares for years afterwards. The prospect of a repeat caesarean filled her with terror but she was determined to be awake to witness the birth of her baby and she wouldn't contemplate a general anaesthetic.

The clinical records validated her account of the events – her blood pressure had indeed dropped dangerously low and tests indicated that the spinal block was very high.

I proposed a simple solution to the patient: 'The problem was caused by an excessive dose in the spinal anaesthetic and obviously you need less than the standard dose. But also we need to make sure you have an adequate dose so you will be comfortable. What I'm going to propose is that we use a combination spinal-epidural anaesthetic. I'm going to put one third of the usual dose in the spinal, we'll let that "cook" for a while, assess the extent of the block, and then top it up using doses in the epidural tubing. We can build up the anaesthetic gently, make sure your blood pressure is stable, and minimize side-effects. How does that sound to you?'

I say to the patient, 'I'm going to put you in charge of what's happening. If you're not OK we'll just stop and figure out what the problem is. If for any reason this isn't going well for you, if you have pain, or you are too distressed, then I can put you to sleep, even half way through the operation. You're in charge of that decision, nobody else can know what you are feeling. You just have to say to me, "Robin, I want to go off to sleep now."'

'I'm going to be here every minute of the case to make sure you're OK. The important thing is that we keep in close communication. If anything is bothering you, I want you to let me know.'

I prepare the patient, 'The spinal anaesthetic doesn't take away all the feeling in your tummy. You are going to feel tugging, pushing and pulling. When the baby is born, the surgeon doesn't make a big cut and just lift the baby out, he's going to squeeze the baby out though a small cut. That's safer for you but it's uncomfortable – you're going to feel someone pushing really hard on the top of your tummy when the baby is being delivered. It's uncomfortable but not painful.'

'There are some side-effects and discomforts you might experience. If that happens, we have some remedies available to make you feel more comfortable. I have them right here on the side. But my intention is that you will feel comfortable and that at the end of the case, all the remedies will still be sitting there unused.'

'You have a wonderful surgeon to care for you. I would choose him to look after my wife or my daughter. We have worked as a team for many years. He's very skilled and quick but he's also gentle. He's very aware you are awake and will be checking with me that you're comfortable.'

These are very deliberate positive suggestions. I'm priming the patient's subconscious mind – a powerful way not only to improve the patient's experience but also to change the physiological responses and to support healing and recovery with minimal complications.

A study at Harvard Medical School randomized patients to receive a pre-op visit from anaesthetists who were deliberately warm, empathetic, positive and reassuring or else the same anaesthetists who adopted a strictly 'clinical' approach to the pre-op visit (Egbert, Battit, Welch, Bartlett, 1964). In the postoperative period, the patients who were primed by the 'positive' anaesthetists had much less pain, consumed only half the amount of morphine, and were discharged from hospital on average 2.7 days earlier!

When I performed the spinal anaesthetic in this patient, I administered only 1ml of anaesthetic, about a third of the normal dose. To my surprise, the patient achieved a perfect block and no epidural top-up was required. The surgery went well and the patient was relaxed, comfortable and joyous in holding her new baby.

I learned something new: that often patients do better with a much smaller dose of the spinal anaesthetic, combined with positive suggestion and compassionate support. I have witnessed a remarkable reduction in patient side-effects with this technique.

My patient was overjoyed. When I saw her the next day she gave me a hug and shed tears. She couldn't believe that her previous trauma could be transformed into a joyous and safe experience. It's one of the most gratifying cases in my career.

Conclusion

When patients spend time in hospital, they remember little of what is said or done but the emotional experience of care stays with them for a lifetime. The culture of healthcare, characterized by high levels of stress, overwork and burnout, erodes the expression of kindness, caring and compassion. Instead, we reward attention to tasks, efficiency and targets. When I've polled health professionals in many countries, the most commonly stated barrier to compassionate care is, "there's no time to care". People blame 'the system' and feel like a helpless cog in the machine.

But even in the most stressed work environment, there are some practitioners who come to work with a smile, have a bubble of calm and stillness around them, always find time for kindness and caring, and seem to be immune to the factors that frustrate the rest of us. What characterizes these practitioners is their deliberate choice of a positive attitude; it gives them enormous power to change the world around them.

The choice is yours.

KEY MESSAGES

- Research shows that medical training is dehumanizing: we lose empathy and tend to adopt a heroic, clinical and detached style of practice.
- Regardless of the rights or wrongs of clinical management, the patients' experience is the only valid measure of care from their perspective.
- We become more compassionate when we adapt our role to become a kind and caring human being first, and a technical expert second.
- Many practitioners suffer from burnout characterized by emotional exhaustion, de-personalization, and loss of a sense of accomplishment. The solution is to reconnect to the heart of your practice and to focus on those parts of your job you can love.

ACTION POINTS

- Even when busy, dispel negative thoughts and try to reflect on the extraordinary privilege of what you do.
- CHOOSE TO LOVE YOUR WORK. Make a deliberate choice about where you focus your attention.
- Learn from others. The performance of health professionals in aspects of kindness, caring, empathy and compassion can develop over time.
- The first greeting with a patient is important. Take care to not only introduce yourself, but your role and intention.
- Remember that simple daily practices that can lift us out of disillusionment and burnout are small acts of kindness, appreciation, gratitude, mindfulness, and self-compassion.

PART II

PRINCIPLES AND THEORIES

12 Human rights principles in maternal health

Diana Bowser and Mande Limbu

Despite recent reductions in rates of maternal and infant mortality (WHO 2012), there is growing evidence that women around the world are subjected to disrespectful and abusive care around the time of childbirth. This chapter summarizes some of the evidence for this, and argues that actions of disrespect and abuse are violations of some of the basic human rights. It examines the health system contexts linked with disrespect and abuse, and the potential solutions that might be inherent in quality improvement approaches. The chapter concludes with an overview of a number of efforts that are currently under way to address disrespect and abuse using a human rights based framework.

Describing the problem

The following story is paraphrased from a woman's account posted on the Bill and Melinda Gates Foundation website website (compiled by Corine Milano). It illustrates some of the issues addressed in this chapter:

> Olutosin was delivering a baby for the first time, as a young woman in Nigeria.[*] Upon preparing for her delivery, she was warned by both her grandmother and her mother about the intense pain of childbirth. What they failed to warn her about was the type of treatment she would receive at the hands of Nigerian healthcare workers that would put her own life and the life of her baby at risk.
>
> Olutosin decided to deliver in a health facility. She arrived at the facility as her labour was progressing. After arriving at the facility, when Olutosin's pain became so intense that she could not bear it any longer, she did not receive any advice on particular techniques that might assist in the delivery or any medications to lessen the pain. Instead the nurses shouted at her 'Shut up! It is time for you to know that a baby's head is bigger than a man's manhood.'
>
> There was no privacy for Olutosin or any of the other women delivering at the same time. They all delivered together and had to share the one bed when it was their turn to deliver. In Olutosin's case, her baby's head crowned before the woman before her was finished using the bed, so the nurse 'sternly warned [her] not to push'. Olutosin tried not to push, but when she could 'not take it any further, [she screamed] and the nurse almost hit [her]'. The nurse yelled 'I told you not to push! No space for you to deliver!'.
>
> Olutosin's labour progressed, but when the baby was finally delivered, it was not breathing. According to Olutosin 'the nurse looked [her] straight in

---

* See the Bill and Melinda Gates website recounting of 'Five Women, Five Stories: Birthing a New Vision for Maternity Care' compiled by Corine Milano: www.impatientoptimists.org/Posts/2013/05/Women-Birth-a-New-Vision-for-Maternity-Care

the face and said disrespectfully, "Witch, you have killed your daughter." She handed the baby to Olutosin's husband and said, "She is a still birth. Your wife killed your child."

This story does have a happy ending, as the baby was subsequently revived. However, the attitudes and behaviours of the staff concerned are clearly a violation of human rights for both the woman and the child. Recently, a USAID funded study has identified the following seven categories of disrespect and abuse: physical abuse, non-consented care, non-confidential care, non-dignified care, discrimination, abandonment of care and financial harassment (Bowser and Hill, 2010). These are further explained in Table 1 below:

Table 1: Categories of Disrespect and Abuse noted in Facility-Based Childbirth, adapted from Bowser and Hill, 2010

Category	Summary of Examples
Physical Abuse	Being beaten, threatened with beating, slapped, rough treatment, pinched, tied down, forceful pushing on the abdomen, pulling a baby out by force, painful stitching without anaesthesia, and withholding of available pain medication when requested.
Non-Consented Care	Absence of patient information and communication processes and/or informed consent for common obstetric procedures, including caesarean sections, episiotomies, hysterectomies, blood transfusions, sterilization, and augmentation of labour.
Non-Confidential Care	Physical lack of privacy (delivering in public view, lack of curtains), lack of privacy related to sensitive patient information such as HIV status, age, marital status, and medical history as well as publicly divulging any of this sensitive information.
Non-Dignified Care	Verbal abuse, intentional humiliation, blaming, scolding, shouting, and intimidation.
Discrimination	Discriminatory behaviour, including non-dignified care and withholding care, from women based on individual characteristics such as race, ethnicity, age, language, HIV/AIDS status, traditional beliefs/preferences, economic status, educational level, and marital status.
Abandonment of Care	Being left alone, unattended, denied evidence-based care, and withholding of moral support and encouragement during and after childbirth.
Financial Harassment	Withholding essential childbirth services until formal or informal payments are made; being held in a health facility after childbirth, sometimes with the newborn child, for failure to pay.

Naming and defining these categories is the first step towards improving the quality of care that women receive surrounding the time of childbirth because it renders disrespectful and abusive behaviours visible, and measurable. They include both those behaviours that can be seen and heard (physical abuse, verbal abuse, abandonment and detention in facilities) as well as more passive forms of violence that overlap closely with human rights violations (non-consented care, non-confidential care, non-dignified care and discrimination).

As well as the immediate harms of such treatment, the experience of, and consequent reputation for, disrespect and abuse in childbirth settings often acts as a deterrent to current and/or future utilization of facility-based childbirth services. This constitutes an important barrier to increasing skilled care utilization and to improving the maternal health outcomes defined by Millennium Development Goal 5, as illustrated in the examples below:

- In Tanzania, a study using a Discrete Choice Experiment found that the most important facility characteristics identified by women as influencing their choice of a facility delivery were provider attitude and drug availability. The authors estimate that improving these facility characteristics would lead to a 43–88% increase in facility delivery (Kruk *et al*, 2009).

- In South Africa, women reported not going for antenatal care because midwives were so rude, meaning that they only attended the local maternity care services when they were in labour (Jewkes, 1998).

- In Nigeria, there is evidence that women do not seek maternal health care at hospitals and clinics due to prior embarrassing experiences or the fear of being humiliated by the healthcare staff (CRR, 2008).

- In Family Care International's report on care-seeking during pregnancy in Kenya (2003) there are numerous anecdotes from women reporting that insults, lack of dignity and respect *'make mothers fearful of seeking care at health facilities'*.

- In Kenya, women report that … *'the nurses don't take care of the patients so we opt for traditional birth attendants. [We] fear going to the hospital'* (Center for Reproductive Rights & Federation of Women Lawyers, Kenya [FIDA], 2007).

- In a study in Peru, many women were reluctant to utilize Emergency Obstetric Care (EmOC) facilities because they felt services paid little attention to their needs and showed little sensitivity toward local culture. After implementation of a programme based on improving infrastructure, staff development, training, supervision and quality, access and use of EmOC increased as well as access to caesarean sections for complicated deliveries (Kayongo *et al*, 2006).

- In Burundi, women who hear of other women being detained in hospitals delay seeking care which can lead to additional complications and risky medical situations (HRW, 2006).
- In the UK, stories of disrespect in childbirth have been reported. Women commonly complain about performance of medical procedures without consent, poor communication (including rudeness, shouting and stereotyping) and even physical abuse during labour (Birthrights, 2013).

Quality of care for women and their newborn infants is also hindered by acts of disrespect and abuse. Improving quality of care is a key in a number of global commitments/action plans such as Every Woman Every Child, Every Newborn Action Plan (2014) and the Post-2015 Development Agenda (ECOSOC, 2014) as well as the new Maternal Health Vision for Action (USAID, 2014).

Finding a solution

There is an association between disrespect and abuse of women during childbirth and weak health systems. Contributions to such system failures include individual and community factors, as well as higher level policy and government factors. Addressing these factors at a systems level demands attention to the promotion and protection of legal and human rights. Some of the mechanisms that can be used include international and regional human rights treaties that highlight explicit and general provisions on women's right to equitable and timely access to good quality, appropriate and non-discriminatory maternity care services. The rights enshrined in these treaties have been specified and interpreted by United Nations treaty monitoring bodies to establish a growing jurisprudence that confirms governments' obligation to guarantee the rights of women during pregnancy and childbirth.

In the context of maternity care, this obligation entails, among other things, governments' commitment to increase the number and improve the quality and conditions of midwives and other health professionals, as well as ensure availability of hospitals, clinics, essential medicines and other supplies. Human rights treaties also affirm the right of every woman to be free from harm and ill treatment (ICCPR, 1966). Applied to maternity care, this right obligates healthcare professionals not to violate pregnant women's right to humane healthcare. More positively, it demands that responsible agents and individuals ensure provision of respectful and compassionate treatment to women during pregnancy and childbirth.

In response to this need, the White Ribbon Alliance (WRA), in collaboration with partners from clinical, educational, research, human rights, and advocacy sectors, has developed the groundbreaking *Respectful Maternity Care Charter: The Universal Rights of Childbearing Women* (WRA, 2011). The seven fundamental maternal rights included in this charter map directly to each of the categories of disrespect and abuse described above. The Charter removes the veil of silence which has shrouded the problem of disrespect and abuse. The Charter has been used as a human rights-based framework and tool for undertaking advocacy, securing policy commitments, increasing visibility of the issue and facilitating dialogue to demand respectful care at all levels: national, regional and local.

Table 2: Mapping of Categories of Disrespect and Abuse to Human Rights

Category	Right of Childbearing Woman
Physical Abuse	Freedom from harm and ill treatment
Non-Consented Care	Respect for choices and preferences
Non-Confidential Care	Right to privacy
Non-Dignified Care	Right to dignity
Discrimination	Freedom from discrimination
Abandonment of Care	Equitable access to care
Financial Harassment	Right to autonomy, self-determination and freedom from coercion

Country-level efforts to address disrespect and abuse have begun over the last several years, focusing on two main areas: human rights-focused policy advocacy, and implementation, as illustrated in the examples below:

- In Nepal, WRA collaborated with the Ministry of Health in Nepal to push for the inclusion of the respectful maternity care rights framework and language into the national Safe Motherhood legislation, thereby ensuring that RMC (Respectful Maternity Care) standards are incorporated into law and in-service curricula for all professional disciplines involved in providing maternal healthcare.
- In Nigeria, WRA is working with the Ministry of Health and other professional bodies to ensure the inclusion of respectful maternity care rights language into professional standard-setting documents. As a result of WRA Nigeria's advocacy, the Ministry of Health agreed to incorporate the rights language in the Life Saving Skills Manual for Midwives in Nigeria. Furthermore, the National Council of Health

approved the Charter as the standard for delivering RMC at all levels of care throughout Nigeria.

- In Malawi, WRA involved the media to put disrespect and abuse in the spotlight as one way of enhancing the quality of maternal healthcare. WRA conducted a journalism contest to build visibility and bring greater attention to the quality of maternal healthcare in Malawi through scale up of quality reporting of positive and negative stories from six districts.

- In Nigeria, WRA is working with Kwara State to provide respectful maternity care to pregnant women in the state. This care will be characterized by quality maternity care where their rights and dignity as women will be protected, through a re-orientation programme for health personnel to ensure that they always abide by the code of conduct and ethics of their different professions.

- In the UK, the maternity education team, supervisors of midwives and governance team at Barking, Havering and Redbridge University Hospitals NHS Trust (BHRUT) joined forces with WRA to incorporate the Respectful Maternity Care Charter into training sessions within maternity services. The sessions are run on a twice-monthly basis and all midwives and obstetric staff are mandated to attend at least once a year.

- Two implementation activities are under way in Kenya and Tanzania, where research protocols have been designed to measure baseline levels of disrespect and abuse in specific communities, implement a programme to decrease disrespect and abuse, and then re-measure the levels of disrespect and abuse after the programme has been implemented.

- In Kenya, the Population Council is implementing a project in five districts in Kenya to examine the issue of disrespect and abuse in maternity care from a number of different perspectives: individual, healthcare provider, community, and policy level (Population Council, 2014).

Conclusion

Application of a rights-based approach to maternity care depends on a well-functioning health system which is responsive to the needs and priorities of women and their families. The right to access quality maternity care can only be realized when health systems use a holistic and people-centred approach where services pay particular attention to women's bodies and minds. A responsive health system which focuses on respect for the dignity of pregnant women, women autonomy and choice, confidentiality, quality of care, and communication, creates an enabling environment for improving interactions women have with the health system, hence advancing their well-being (Gostin, 2003). The veil of silence has been broken. The need for compassionate maternity care that is founded in respect and dignity is now starkly evident. This should mean that, in future, there are far more birth stories in which mother and baby are alive and well and where mother and baby have both received the most dignified and respectful treatment.

KEY MESSAGES

- The disrespect and abuse of women in childbirth is widespread, and occurs in all countries of the world.
- Addressing disrespect and abuse requires an understanding of the drivers on many different levels as well as a human rights-based approach. This can happen at the individual level, the community level, through policy and advocacy.
- Policies and interventions to maximize respectful and dignified care can be effective.

ACTION POINTS

- Each individual maternity care practitioner, service provider and service funder needs to think 'what can I do in my everyday job to reduce disrespect and abuse for mothers and babies', and to put the resulting solutions into action every day.
- Researchers, funders and commissioners of research need to design, commission, fund and implement studies to:
  - understand the mechanisms by which disrespect and abuse deter women from using health facilities for childbirths
  - understand the reasons for, and to measure the extent of, disrespect and abuse surrounding the time of childbirth
  - maximize respectful and dignified maternity care.
- Professional bodies must incorporate RMC in standard setting documents. For example, the WRA Respectful Maternity Care Charter can be embedded in professional bodies' regulatory standards and/or guidelines, as well as training curricula for all health workers providing maternity care.
- Communities need to be mobilized to address disrespect and abuse and demand their right to RMC, through a range of routes, including local media.
- Governments need to increase advocacy, policy and resource allocation at the national and sub-national levels, and to ensure that maternal health – related laws, policies and plans address disrespect and abuse and include maternity-specific provisions.

13 How kindness, warmth, empathy and support promote the progress of labour: a physiological perspective

Kerstin Uvnäs Moberg

The objective of this chapter is to demonstrate how friendly, supportive and competent maternity care workers may facilitate the progress of labour by triggering optimal neuroendocrine and physiological mechanisms involved in birth. The role of oxytocin release in response to touch, stroking, light pressure and warmth and in response to analogous positive mental stimuli will be highlighted.

In order to facilitate the understanding of how environmental and mental factors may influence the process of birth some basic physiological mechanisms involved in the regulation of birth will be described.

Role of oxytocin and the autonomic nervous system during labour

Birth is an innate spontaneous process. The body 'knows' how to transfer the fetus from the womb to the outside world. A multitude of neuro-hormonal mechanisms stimulate and integrate the different aspects of the birth process.

Oxytocin plays an important role in this respect, as it is released in pulses into the circulation to stimulate uterine contractions. When the infant's head presses against the cervix of the uterus sensory nerves (the hypogastric and pelvic nerves) are activated. The neurogenic impulses transmit information to the SON (supraoptic nucleus) and PVN (paraventricular nucleus), via the spinal cord and the brainstem, and more oxytocin is released (the Fergusson reflex) and in this way the contractions are reinforced.

Oxytocin is, however, also released from oxytocinergic nerves within the brain during labour. By stimulation of oxytocin release from parvocellular neurons from the PVN, pain threshold is increased, some aspects of social interactive behaviours are stimulated, and stress levels and autonomic nervous tone are modulated. Pain sensation, emotion and psychological status are therefore inter-related with oxytocin release.

Both the parasympathetic and the sympathetic nervous system influence the pattern of uterine contractions. Stimulation of the parasympathetic nerves that innervate the uterus (the pelvic nerve) gives rise to uterine contractions and at the same time uterine blood flow is increased. Stimulation of the sympathetic nerves (the hypogastric nerve) on the other hand induces prolonged uterine contractions and at the same time uterine blood flow is decreased.

Link between oxytocin and autonomic nervous tone

Interestingly there are important anatomical and functional connections between the oxytocin system and the parasympathetic and the sympathetic nervous system. Oxytocinergic fibres emanating in the PVN project to autonomic nervous centres in the brain stem and spinal cord, where oxytocin shifts the balance in the autonomic nervous system towards an increased parasympathetic and a decreased sympathetic nervous tone.

Extremely long oxytocinergic nerves originating in the PVN project all the way down via the spinal cord to the parasympathetic nervous plexa in the sacral region. These fibres connect with postsynaptic cholinergic nerve fibres, which innervate the uterus and which stimulate uterine contractions.

Several oxytocinergic mechanisms participate in both milk ejection and uterine contractions

In order to really understand the interplay between circulating effects of oxytocin and the activity in the autonomic nervous system, it may be of help to compare how these two regulatory mechanisms interplay during labour and milk ejection.

As is well known, oxytocin not only stimulates uterine muscles in connection with labour it also stimulates contractions of the myoepithelial cells in the mammary gland in connection with milk ejection during breastfeeding. In fact oxytocin does not only contract muscles, it may also relax muscles to facilitate labour and breastfeeding. In addition nervous mechanisms, in particular parasympathetic and sympathetic nervous tone, will influence the effects caused by circulating oxytocin.

These hormonal effects exerted by oxytocin are facilitated by nervous mechanisms in several ways. Suckling triggers local neurogenic reflexes (axon reflexes), which facilitate the milk ejection reflex by relaxing the muscles of the milk duct sphincters, thereby 'opening the doors' for an increased milk flow.

External factors such as stressors inhibit milk ejection by stimulating the sympathetic nerves, which then work to contract the milk ducts, and inhibit the let down reflex. Infant suckling, and touching of the breast stimulate afferent sensory nerves, which inhibit the sympathetic tone. In this way stress-induced contraction of the milk ducts is counteracted by infant behaviours. Oxytocin is then released within the brain in response to suckling to induce an anxiolytic effect and to reduce stress levels including sympathetic nervous tone. These effects contribute to the facilitation of milk let down.

As noted above, an important aspect of the oxytocin-related effect spectrum during labour is that oxytocin appears to induce two different hormonal effects: it contracts the uterus, but it also takes part in relaxation of the birth canal, which will of course facilitate expulsion of the fetus. This double effect is completely in analogy with the dual effects that oxytocin exerts in connection with milk ejection: it contracts the myoepithelial cells and relaxes the milk ducts. The process of milk ejection is from a basic functional point of view very similar to the fetal ejection (Fergusson) reflex.

Oxytocin is, however, not only released into the circulation in response to activation of the Fergusson reflex. It is also released from nerves projecting from the PVN to areas where the autonomic nervous activity is controlled. In this way the long oxytocin-containing nervous fibres, which travel within the spinal cord to reach the parasympathetic plexa in the sacral region and which contribute to the stimulation of uterine muscles, are activated. The parasympathetic nervous activity promotes the effects of oxytocin on the progress of labour and the sympathetic nervous system inhibits.

Where do kindness and caring come in?

Pleasant sensory stimulation of the skin during birth (touch, stroking, warmth and light pressure) benefits the process of birth in an analogous way. By decreasing sympathetic nervous tone and by increasing parasympathetic nervous tone the progress of birth is facilitated, as the autonomic nervous system participates in the regulation of uterine contractions. Decreased levels of anxiety and stress in response to oxytocin released within the brain area will also promote the process of labour as the balance in the autonomic nervous tone will be shifted from sympathetic to parasympathetic tone.

The process of labour is, therefore not completely automatic, as it is influenced by environmental factors and the mother's state of mind. The mother needs to feel safe and protected and so the birthing place must be perceived as safe and welcoming, since it is known that oxytocin release and uterine contractions stop in an environment that is perceived by the mother to be 'dangerous'. Oxytocin is simply not released under these circumstances, as, from an evolutionary perspective, it is risky to give birth in unfamiliar surroundings that feel unsafe. The onset of labour may be delayed, or active labour may be prolonged, if the pregnant woman is stressed or afraid. This may be due to psychological factors such as previous memories of a traumatic birth, or to frightening stories about birth she may have heard, or it may be a result of growing stressors subsequent to a cycle of a birth that is long, painful and doesn't progress.

Also the type of interaction between the individuals present during birth (relatives, midwives, doctors or doulas) and the birthing woman is of importance. In the presence of a maternity care worker who is very controlling, un-empathic or even rude, the birth process is slowed down because the labouring woman becomes afraid and stressed.

In all these negative stress-related situations oxytocin release may be decreased. Also the balance between parasympathetic and sympathetic nervous tone may shift. When the activity of the sympathetic nervous system is prolonged, painful and less 'efficient' contractions may be induced and in addition the circulation to the uterus might be restricted.

Impact of medical interventions on oxytocin production

Although clinical and pharmacological interventions are important tools in intrapartum care where true pathology exists, the ever-broadened range of indications for these interventions and the enormous increase in the use of them may induce unwanted effects. For example, epidural analgesia and infusions of exogenous oxytocin may interfere with the birth process itself, and therefore, become the cause of rather than the solution to problems in labour, especially when they interfere with the release of endogenous oxytocin. In this case, the consequence may be a restriction in the development of oxytocin-mediated physiological and behavioural adaptations, which would usually occur during mother and infant in spontaneous physiological labour, or which might otherwise be triggered via skin-to-skin contact after birth. For example, the enhanced social interaction between mother and infant normally observed after birth may not develop as well as it should, and some intrapartum maternal, physiological adaptations that have evolved to facilitate breastfeeding in the mother may not take place.

When mothers feel safe and supported the progress of labour is facilitated

Home-like setting If the place where a woman gives birth looks familiar and welcoming and if light and sound are dampened, the progress of labour will be better, because the function of the physiological mechanisms involved in birth will be optimized. In particular, when melatonin levels rise, the sympathetic nervous tone is decreased.

Friendly and supportive staff It is increasingly evident that the attitude and behaviour of other humans who are present at birth matters. A positive, friendly and empathic treatment by the staff or other people who are present at birth can optimize the hormonal and endocrine responses in the mother that can make birth quicker and less painful, and that can change it into a more positive experience. In the longer term, mothers who have experienced this may feel happier, and their interaction with their newborn may be optimized.

The following section examines the physiological factors that might underpin these empirical observations.

Sensory stimulation of the skin

Noxious stimulation If the skin is hurt or exposed to strong stimuli (noxious stimulation), certain types of nerve fibres that originate in the skin are activated that causes awareness of the pain. In addition, a stress response is induced, in which blood pressure and cortisol levels rise. This is a direct consequence of activation of nerves, as it also occurs in animals that are anaesthetized and therefore not afraid of the experimental situation. The neuro-endocrine and behavioural reactions to noxious stimulation are integrated in the hypothalamus and in the brainstem.

Non-noxious stimulation In contrast, if the skin is exposed to soothing stimuli, by stroking, touch, light pressure and a pleasantly warm temperature, an anti-stress response is induced, and stress levels, as measured by blood pressure, heart rate and cortisol levels, decrease. In addition, social interactive behaviours may be induced, further reducing psychological anxiety and, consequently, perception of pain. This leads to an enhanced sense of wellbeing.

Oxytocin released from oxytocinergic nerves originating in the PVN, which project to many important regulatory areas in the brain, plays an important controlling function in this reaction pattern (the so called 'calm and connect' response, that has been contrasted to the better known stress response of 'fight or flight'). In the context of already high oxytocin levels, the oxytocinergic pathways projecting from the PVN to the brainstem are enhanced, allowing for even more oxytocin to be released. This means that oxytocin release in response to sensory stimulation of the skin is facilitated if oxytocin levels are already high, as, for example, when in the presence of a kind and friendly person. Given that this response can be mediated by what has been termed 'therapeutic touch', physical closeness and skin to skin contact between the labouring woman and her caregivers during labour, and between the woman and her infant during breastfeeding, is an important part of this physiological process.

Link between emotions and neuroendocrine reactions caused by mental processes and somatosensory stimulation

Many people believe that sensory and mental stimuli operate via completely different nervous and neuroendocrine mechanisms, but this is not the case. Experiences created from the environment (or thoughts and memories) induce feelings and neuroendocrine and physiological effects in much the same way as does information from the skin mediated by sensory nerves.

To experience something dangerous and threatening or to think of such things basically gives rise to the same stress reactions (variants of the fight and flight reaction), as does damage to the body. Feelings (or perhaps sensations is a better word) and associated neuroendocrine and physiological reactions induced via nerves that innervate the skin are, from an evolutionary perspective, older than those induced by mental stimuli. As the function of the CNS and the frontal cortex developed, experiences mediated via higher senses (e.g. vision), as well as memories of previous experiences, have become increasingly more important regulators of basic behavioural and neuro-endocrine reaction patterns.

Interestingly the terminology of some of the most basic mental feelings (feeling good, supported, held and warm or feeling bad, alone and cold) actually mirror the modalities of information that can by induced following stimulation of sensory nerves from the skin.

In this context it is also of interest to point out that the skin and the nervous system are related from a developmental point of view. Actually the central nervous system develops as an invagination of the ectoderm, which also gives rise to the skin in the embryo. The sense of touch develops first and later on, as the fetus grows, all the other senses develop as invaginations of the skin. No wonder that the skin not only acts like a barrier to the exterior world, but retains an important role as a sensory organ connecting the external world and the CNS.

Link to kindness

Since both oxytocin and parasympathetic nervous tone play important roles during birth, any stimuli that promote oxytocin release and parasympathetic nervous tone will promote the process of labour. Pleasant stimulation of the skin (e.g. touch, stroking, light pressure and warm temperature) activates sensory nerves and represents one mechanism by which oxytocin release and increased activation of the parasympathetic and decreased activity of the sympathetic nervous system can be achieved.

This may explain why bathing in pleasantly warm water promotes labour. The warm bath transmits warmth and exerts a light pressure on the skin of the birthing mother. Oxytocin release, and in particular the parasympathetic tone, two important mechanisms in the promotion of labour, will be increased. In addition, the release of oxytocin in the brain may exert a pain-relieving effect. For the same reason touching and other types of pleasant stimulation of the mother's skin induced by the staff will promote birth.

It is important to note that this process operates for staff as well as for labouring women. In order to transmit kindness and support to mothers, staff and other people who are present during the birth must feel calm and confident themselves.

Conclusion

The dynamic interconnection between psychological and emotional responses to labour and birth, and the neuro-hormonal activity that is necessary to ensure that labour and birth progresses optimally, is only recently being explored in depth. The essential role of oxytocin in the process of uterine contractions has been understood for some time, but evidence is now emerging that oxytocin acts on a range of different maternal systems in complex and highly nuanced ways. Applying this knowledge to practice indicates it is vital that maternity care staff or any other people present during birth are perceived as kind, empathic and supportive by the mother giving birth. Labouring women not only listen to the spoken word, they read the facial expressions and the body language, and they listen to the tone of voice in order to unconsciously make a judgement as to whether the person is friendly, and to be trusted, or not. In the presence of kind people oxytocin is released into the circulation and the brain and the progress of birth is facilitated. If the mother doesn't feel safe and welcomed no oxytocin is released and stress levels including sympathetic nervous tone are increased. In addition the sensory input from the skin, which should give rise to further oxytocin release, is blocked. All of those attending labouring women should have an understanding of these processes, and of the potential consequences of the emotional and psychological environment in which women labour and give birth.

KEY MESSAGES

- Labouring women not only listen to the spoken word, they read the facial expressions and the body language, and they listen to the tone of voice in order to unconsciously make a judgement as to whether the person is friendly, and to be trusted, or not.
- An increasing number of studies are demonstrating the dynamic inter-

connection between psychological and emotional states during labour, and maternal neuro-hormonal activity.

- Oxytocin acts on a range of different maternal systems in complex and highly nuanced ways.
- Oxytocin production in labour is up-regulated by a range of factors, including therapeutic touch, and the presence of kind and caring attendants.
- Oxytocin is down-regulated when the environment is cold and unwelcoming, and in the presence of disrespectful or abusive behaviours and attitudes.

ACTION POINTS

- All staff attending women in labour need to keep up to date with the current and emerging evidence on the role of oxytocin in labour and birth.
- All staff attending women in labour need to be aware that their attitudes and behaviours can have measurable effects on maternal production of oxytocin, and, therefore, on labour progress.
- Those designing and providing services, including policy makers and managers, should ensure that staff can work in an environment that maximises their wellbeing and, therefore, the optimal experience and progress of labour and birth for the women they are attending.

14 Spirituality, compassion and maternity care

Jenny Hall

In the United Kingdom there is an expectation that midwifery care will involve recognition of the centrality of the woman and her family and a holistic, whole person approach to care. Holistic principles include the importance of spiritual care, an aspect that remains elusive in the midwifery literature (Hall, 2013), despite the depth of understanding for those at the end of life. Embedded in the NHS constitution is the concept of 'value based care' where 'everyone counts' that includes the centrality of the service user, care that is respectful and ensures dignity, which aims to improve lives, demonstrates commitment to quality care and is compassionate. The purpose of this discussion is to consider the links between the concepts of spirituality and compassionate care.

The spiritual nature of birth

Birth is a transformative process of life where women move from one state of being into another. It is therefore not surprising that women consider birth to be a spiritual event. For example:

> The experience itself is so different from anything you ever experience except when you're having birth, so in that respect, I think it's a spiritual experience, just as any other rites of passage... it's an experience that you never forget... [It's] spiritual and significant...because of the feelings that you have, the lessons that you learn, the insights in relation to the experience. (Klassen, 2001:94)

It is, however, surprising that there has been limited exploration of the spiritual nature of birth. Midwives also care for babies and in reality some babies are not born to live. Care therefore should include the recognition of the spiritual nature of the unborn/newborn and a need to treat babies with gentleness and kindness, promoting values for humanity. In a recent study of the meaning of midwifery the midwife participants related spiritual care to the 'art' of midwifery; acknowledges individual religious belief; recognizes women's individual resources and is intuitive (Hall, 2011). Midwives consequently are viewing their role as spiritual and this is based in the context of relationship with the woman and family. The factor of relationship is included in the suggestion that:

> Spiritual care begins with encouraging human contact in compassionate relationship, and moves in whatever direction need requires.' (NHS Education for Scotland, 2010)

Compassion and spirituality

The indication is that compassionate care and spiritually based care are inextricably linked.

Contemporary definitions of compassionate care call it 'sympathetic consciousness of others' distress' with the added proviso that the concern is acted upon. It implies recognition of the other being of worth, of a depth of care that goes beyond a simple professional relationship. It is empathetic and loving. Such depth of care is highlighted by the principles of '*caritas*' (Lundmark, 2007; Watson, 2008), which appears to be an ability to care from 'higher/deeper dimensions of humanity' and 'human to human connections' (Watson, 2008).

This intensity of relationship is grounded in historical western-based midwifery practice. The midwife was the 'woman that women went to'; midwives were chosen by the community to be alongside those suffering at the end of life and at the start. In a sense they were 'called' by others, and they had a vocation. In the latter years nursing and midwifery were based in a 'religious life' where midwives were expected to be dedicated in service to the role. There was sacrifice of themselves where they were not expected to be married or have children and based in the community, on call to everyone at all times. They were 'known', and in being 'known', trusted and in relationship with the woman and family. The Old English term of '*midwyf*', meaning 'with woman', illustrates the 'being with' link with compassionate care. The midwife stands alongside with integrity and honesty in the relationship.

In modern times there has been an increase in technological intervention and a move away from relationship, with the midwife's role becoming more based in the science, as opposed to art. However, it could be argued that women in more complicated situations might need more spiritual care and therefore more demonstration of compassion.

Victor Frankl, a psychiatrist writing of his experience in a concentration camp, stated that: *'Man is not destroyed by suffering; he is destroyed by suffering without meaning'* (Frankl, 1984)

This is not to say that women during pregnancy and birth 'suffer' to the intensity of Frankl's experience but women have a different intensity of emotions and pain and may also experience illness. In the role of the compassionate, alongside person, midwives can and do bring meaning to the process of birth. To suggest that women may also be destroyed by the suffering they endure is a truth where women are diagnosed with post-traumatic stress, even after a so-called 'normal' birth. In these situations the potential lack of compassion by midwives could be recognized.

Midwives in the study mentioned previously saw their role as being part of their identity, or who they are (Hall, 2012). However, midwives should also recognize their motivation for the role they have chosen. There is a suggestion that our choice to be within the caring professions is linked to the desire to deal with problems 'or unresolved hopes, hurts and fears from the past' (Barratt and Campling, 2011). In order to provide compassionate care the individual needs to be self-aware in recognition of motivations but also to recognize the effects of constantly giving in challenging work situations without support as this may lead to being burnt out and unable to give (Yoder, 2010; Mollart *et al,* 2011). Spiritual compassionate care also relates to the self-worth and needs of the carer.

It is also evident that the individual midwife is not the only factor in the difficulty in providing compassionate care. Others have suggested that the organization of care is significant in enabling an appropriate attitude of care (Crawford *et al,* 2014). The move of midwifery to be more hospital-focused with reduced staffing and less time to provide care does not lead to ease in provision of the art of midwifery (Hall, 2012). It is appropriate to suggest that there would be a greater ability to provide spiritual compassionate care in an environment where midwives are working in a way where they are able to build up a relationship with women, as they are educated to do; where policies reflect the expectations of their role; where they have time to provide the care they expect to give and in a physical environment which is aesthetically beautiful as well as comfortable to work in.

Conclusion

The current move to return to values of dignity, care and compassion across healthcare indicates recognition that these have been lost somewhere. It is apparent that these values are linked to spiritually based care, which suggests some notice should be taken of deeper levels of practice. It is evident that for many cultures birth remains a 'rite of passage' yet in the western world there remains a tendency to focus on physical care. In order to increase compassion there is a need to revisit the art of midwifery and the structures and organizations in which it is placed. In addition, and perhaps to a greater level, the start of life should be viewed as a life-changing and precious event that is meaningful and significant to women and families but also to the midwives who care. It is not thought of as 'just a job' but a role that is close to the heart of humanity, at the borders of life and death, where the values of trust, love and compassion are real and significant (Hall, 2013).

KEY MESSAGES

- Birth is a transformative event that is regarded as spiritual.
- Compassionate care is viewed as an aspect of spiritual care.
- Women with complicated births also require spiritually based care.
- Consideration should be made of models of care and environment of care.
- Compassionate care also includes the midwife's self-awareness of her needs.

ACTION POINTS

- Remember that birth is a transformative meaningful process for the woman and her family.
- Treat the woman and baby with gentleness and kindness, remembering the humanity of each as individuals.
- Focus on the holistic needs compassionately of those with complicated pregnancies.
- Explore how the models of care you work in can be altered to improve compassionate spiritually based care.
- Consider how the environment you work in can be improved to be more welcoming to women.
- Consider how the working environment can be improved for staff to encourage spiritual care.

15 Stop the fear and embrace birth

Hannah Dahlen and Kathryn Gutteridge

As one of us has noted in a previous publication: 'We cannot hope to begin to deal with women's fear of childbirth unless we are willing to examine our own, and recognize how we can and do contribute to women's fear.' *(Dahlen, 2010) Fear of childbirth in women has been extensively studied, but much less has been written about health provider fear, and about how this fear may impact on women and birth. Fear in maternity care has become transcribed into our DNA, so to speak, passed on from health provider to heath provider, and most worryingly from health provider to women. Our birth environments also construct fear in a way that affects both the expectations and experiences of childbearing women, and the practice of health professionals. The most urgent message in the roar behind the silence should be to stop the fear now! To do this, though, we need to turn our focus towards the way we see birth, and onto the environments we provide for women to birth in. To address these issues, Hannah begins this chapter by examining the culture of fear, with a particular focus on health professionals. Kathryn then goes on to explore the role of environment in affecting not only childbearing women, but maternity care professionals as well. We both then discuss ways of shifting the focus from fear to compassionate care for all those providing and receiving maternity services.*

Examining the culture of fear (Hannah)

While significant attention has been focused on women's fear in the contemporary scientific literature (Nieminen *et al*, 2009; Rouhe *et al*, 2012) and media (Morris and McInerney, 2010) there has been less attention focused on the fears of health providers and how they may be impacting on women's fear (Dahlen, 2010; Otely, 2011; Regan and Liaschenko, 2007). In Powell Kennedy's (2004) qualitative study examining midwives beliefs about normal birth some of the midwives reported that when they became fearful while caring for women giving birth they were less able to care optimally for the woman and they reported that their anxiety may have impacted negatively on the birth outcome (Powell Kennedy and Shannon, 2004). In these rare examples of honesty we begin to see the question raised: how do we contribute to women's fear when it comes to childbirth?

What do midwives fear?

A recent study we undertook in Australia and New Zealand looked at the top fears midwives hold when it comes to their job. Over 739 midwives' fears were analyzed and eight categories were found, including death of a baby, and missing something that causes harm. They also talked about the fear of being watched and criticized (Dahlen and Caplice, 2014). In another Australian study we undertook, midwives were asked to look at a photo of a woman in labour that potentially elicited multiple interpretations, and they were asked a series of open questions about the possible story behind the photograph and how they would hypothetically provide care. Midwives described the conflicting contexts of childbirth they worked in, and how, as labour progressed, they felt pressure to 're-linquish' or compromise their desire to support women to give birth as normally as possible (Copeland *et al,* 2013).

The problem with fear is that, while it can be protective and important for survival, it can also alter behaviour and thinking. Physiologically fear can leave indelible memory traces, with researchers showing that even after a fear inducing stimulus has been extinguished, the brain retains a changed pattern of neuronal firing in response to that stimulus (LeDoux *et al,* 1989; Quirk *et al,* 1995). This means that midwives working in environments where there are high levels of fear, and where they feel they are under surveillance, are potentially being primed to be even more fearful.

A risk approach or a safety approach?

Managing risk is not the same as facilitating safety (Dahlen, 2014). Taking a risk approach is like telling your child who is learning to ride a bike, not to hit the wall you have spotted in the distance. As their eye locks onto the wall ahead and they begin to concentrate on avoiding it they are no longer riding safely; their joy decreases, their anxiety increases and the chances of riding into the wall or deviating off the path escalate, because they are so focused on the wall. Even if they manage to avoid the wall, what joy has there been in the ride and why ride if you get no joy from it? In maternity care we are constantly sending the message to women and to each other that we need to 'avoid the wall'.

Under this paradigm the psychological, social, cultural and spiritual factors that may enhance safety and are that what make us human are hard to quantify and so are ignored (Dahlen, 2014). It is hardly surprising then that ignoring these important 'other' aspects of safety is leading increasingly to traumatized women and dehumanised care, and this creates other risks (for example freebirth) that as health providers we tend to blame on irresponsible women, being blind to how we are failing some women badly (Jackson *et al,* 2012).

Learning to dance in the grey zone

Over 2000 years ago the Greek philosopher Aristotle talked about virtue as consisting of choosing the *mean* ('the golden mean') between two extremes (Woods, 1982). For example, if one faces mortal danger Aristotle says courage consists of choosing the *mean* between recklessness on one hand and cowardice on the other. Aristotle proposes the *mean* and the *good*, is feeling [or acting] at the right time, about the right things in relation to the right people and for the right reason (Woods, 1982). Choosing the mean consists of applying logic and taking a case-by-case approach. Aristotle emphasized the importance of relationships to give us the opportunity for goodness and happiness and the need for rationality and contemplation. In maternity care I have called this '*dancing in the grey zone between normality and risk*' (Dahlen, 2012). Most of maternity care, if we are really honest, is grey. Dancing in the grey zone makes us responsive, vigilant and opens up the possibility of birth. Wayne Dyer said, '*When you dance, your purpose is not to get to a certain place on the floor. It's to enjoy each step along the way*'. It's time to bring enjoyment back into maternity care provision. Surely that enjoyment begins with seeing women as being full of capacity not full of catastrophe.

Relationship-based care

The best way to safely *dance in the grey zone* is by moving towards relationship-based care. Developing partnerships with women leads us to become invested in the care we give, share the responsibility and see remarkable outcomes for women and babies (Sandall *et al*, 2013; Schindler *et al*, 2004). Maternity care staff act, talk and interact differently with women they know and are invested in (Teate *et al*, 2013). If we focused on safety and not risk, on relationship-based care, not system-based care, we could make maternity care safer for everyone (women, health professionals and organizations) (Dahlen, 2014). Learning to trust in women and birth is a sure way for women to trust in themselves and their capacity to give birth. As Karl Menninger said, '*fears are educated into us and can, if we wish, be educated out*'. By creating environments of trust where relationship-based care is prioritized, where birth is revered, not feared, and where midwives and other maternity care staff are encouraged to draw on their knowledge, skills and intuition in consultation with women, we will start to turn the culture of fear into one of trust and towards facilitating true safety in its broadest sense (physical, psychological, cultural and spiritual).

Tips for helping maternity care staff deal with fear

- Identify what you are fearful of.
- Share your fear(s) with someone you trust.
- Take responsibility for them – most are a creation in your mind.
- When you are faced directly with what you fear, consciously take slow breaths to slow everything down, so that you can think your way out of the situation.
- Observe yourself talking: practise stopping negative thoughts.
- Use positive visualization.
- Have a cup of tea.
- Knit or crochet at births – it reduces adrenaline.
- Do an obstetric emergency skills course like ALSO.
- Write about your specific fear(s) and reflect on them.
- Centre yourself with affirmations such as trust in the process.
- Be sceptical when others fuel fear; gather information, think carefully.
- Beware the language of fear as it has many forms.
- Remember the loudest voice in the room usually comes from the most frightened person.
- Balance your fear with faith in human female physiology.
- Reassure your colleagues that we can reassure women that birth is normal.
- Facilitate women to trust in their ability to handle the outcome, whatever it may be.
- Retell positive stories about birth to each other and to women.
- Most importantly, shed your fears after each encounter and do not carry them to the next birth.

First published in *What do Midwives Fear?* (Dahlen and Caplice, 2014)

Creating environments of trust (Kathryn)

Over a century ago Florence Nightingale recognized the value and healing qualities of the environment in harmonization with professional knowledge. She noted that '*what nursing has to do… is to put the patient in the best condition for nature to act upon him*' (Selanders, 2010). This sentiment seems perfectly sensible and not out of date at all in our modern maternity environments; however, it is increasingly lost in modern maternity care provision.

Giving birth is a unique experience for women; even the same woman having subsequent births will have different experiences of her labours. The irony is that whilst labour and birth for most women is expected to be normal and straightforward, in women's accounts and memories it is far from that (Simkin, 1992). What is going wrong in the journeys women make to motherhood and what is the dynamic between the woman and her environment that generates fear?

Wagner (2001) invites women to think about the choices they make for their labours and to take responsibility for the people and the place in which their birth will take place (Wagner, 2001). Working within women's communities restores a balance between health provider and women. In my experience in midwifery, it is easy to see a respectful relationship between both woman and midwife where a sense of trust and resonance develops like perfectly paired dancers. There is mutuality in how one cares for the other.

In general healthcare, hospital environments that have dedicated attention to the social and spiritual qualities for patients are as yet poorly researched and little understood. However, a systematic review has reported that positive effects were found where wards are designed to capture maximum sunlight, where patients have access to windows, where pleasant odours are used, and where seating arrangements allow for the development of relationships between patients (Dijkstra *et al*, 2006). Attributes such as music and space were less clearly beneficial.

Over the last three decades in the United Kingdom interest has increased in defining the optimum birth environment. A realization that clinical settings may have a harmful effect on the labour and birth is now well documented, and women are exercising their choices with that knowledge (Hodnett *et al*, 2012; Hodnett *et al*, 2013; Walsh and Gutteridge, 2011). Policies and reports that support less clinical settings are well established and embedded within most modern maternity services and feature regularly in political documents (Department of Health UK, 2014).

There is something very different about the way labour and birth unfolds in a home environment when compared to a hospital setting (Gutteridge, 2013). When at home a woman in early labour is mobile and active, and she unconsciously prepares her own surroundings to meet the changing needs of her labouring body. She is more often than not excited rather than fearful; her homely surroundings, which are familiar to her, with family nearby, are not intrusive or distracting (Walsh and Gutteridge, 2011). Hammond *et al*, (2013) refer to the effect that birthing space has upon midwives' behaviour and how different environments influence their performance with women (Hammond *et al*, 2013). The space and time to watch and wait for labour to progress in its most natural state is limited within clinical hospital settings (Gutteridge, 2013).

The incremental production of oxytocin takes the woman through her labour whilst she also produces increasingly higher levels of endorphins that can soothe her discomfort. Movement also aids the process, and women in more home-like environments can be observed to move around to aid their discomfort. This process is much less evident in clinical settings, where beds are placed centrally in labour rooms, leading women to become recumbent and passive (Priddis *et al*, 2012; Priddis *et al*, 2011). Davis-Floyd and Cheyney (2009) noted that in home-like birth environments '*They [women] labored and birthed in upright positions using instinctive knowledge to expand the size of the pelvis, capitalize on gravity, and to maximize the efficiency of the abdominal muscles needed for pushing* ' (Davis-Floyd and Cheyney, 2009).

Sutton (2000) noted that women in labour with fetuses in a posterior presentation adopt 'all-fours' positions or to raise a corresponding leg at the height of a contraction (Sutton, 2000). Somehow women understand the needs of their bodies during labour, and this triggers physiological responses to their discomfort that, in turn, enable labour to progress.

Learning from end of life care

Over the last 25 years end of life care has transformed care for the dying. Palliative care has focused on providing appropriate environments and supporting the individual's personal needs. The hospice movement has worked increasingly hard to provide resources and accommodation that cares for the sickest patients in our society. All efforts are centred around the incorporation of the beauty of nature, natural light, and the use of space. A high degree of energy is put into maintaining dignity and privacy. This seems a perfect formula for meeting the needs of the dying and their families where spirituality and peace is valued in equal parts to clinical and pharmacological treatments. How is this so different from the needs of those yet to be born and the women who will give birth to them?

Where midwives and other maternity caregivers are comfortable in their practice and in their ability to provide woman-centred care designed to optimize women's capacity to birth physiologically, they become quietly confident and skilled in their art; women who receive care from them are able to respond to all of the positive influencers that will progress their labour. This is demonstrated in all elements of care, clinical outcomes and satisfaction levels at Serenity and Halcyon Birth Centres (Gutteridge, 2014). Bringing about a change in service for women and their caregivers has seen a consistent improvement in clinical outcomes at all levels, reduction in staff sickness and vacancies. Satisfaction levels are above 92%.

Pathologizing birth is harmful: it holds women prisoner, affecting their experiences and memories for eternity. It is the task of midwives and obstetricians to reverse this trend and place birth where it belongs, within the family's grasp rather than starting from a position of risk.

Plato said *'We can easily forgive a child who is afraid of the dark; the real tragedy of life is when men are afraid of the light'*. We have the solutions to the problem; we now need to show courage in applying these.

Conclusion

Alexander Solzhenitsyn (1918–2008) asked, *'If one is forever cautious, can one remain a human being?'* It is time to reclaim our humanity in maternity care before it is too late, not by throwing caution to the wind but by understanding that the attitudes, culture and environments surrounding birth can create fear. In this chapter we have look at the fear paralyzing modern maternity care providers and we have placed the maternity culture and the environments in which we care for women under the microscope. We have joined the roar behind the silence with a cry to stop fear and to embrace birth.

KEY MESSAGES

- Health professionals need to examine how their fears may impact on women.
- Balance your fear with faith in human female physiology.
- Learning to trust in women and birth is a sure way for women to trust in themselves and their capacity to give birth.
- Birth environments impact on both women and maternity care staff.
- Relationships of trust between women and midwives and other maternity care providers help reduce fear and facilitate normal birth.
- Birth environments such as home birth and free standing midwife led units for low-risk women impact on the way women and midwives act.

ACTION POINTS

- Don't ignore your fears. Explore them and address them.
- Our fears tell us where we need to develop skills and confidence, so if you have a particular fear, for example shoulder dystocia, then set up ways and means of overcoming what underlies that fear (for example, attend an obstetric emergencies course.)
- Most importantly consciously work to shed your fears before you carry them to the next birth you attend.
- Think about how you can change the environment you work in to reduce fear and to increase the capacity for compassionate care for yourself, your colleagues and the women you are working with.

16 How environment and context can influence capacity for kindness

Mavis Kirkham

I don't think anyone came into midwifery in order to be unkind and to process women, or, if need be, to bully them through a system. I have seen generations of students enter midwifery with the highest aspirations and motivation to serve childbearing families. Yet the context of clinical care in the National Health Service (NHS) so often serves to knock these aspirations out of them as they struggle to cope with the demands placed upon them. This chapter addresses some of the issues that contextualize the call for kindness and compassion in midwifery, and, by extension, to other maternity care workers.

Time is money

Kindness involves a degree of openness and listening, which the market-driven NHS and its workers literally cannot afford. At the highest level, a model of healthcare has been chosen which squeezes out compassion. Yet the practitioners, not the model, are blamed for unkindness. There are all sorts of acts of kindness which only take moments, but time is money and moments add up across the working day. True compassion involves listening, making ourselves available and being able to do something about what we hear. That does not fit in a highly structured, fragmented and standardized service.

Midwives often feel guilty because they cannot work harder and longer and because it is impossible to be consistently kind in the face of a system which unkindly treats them as cogs in a machine, rather than as people. Such guilt hurts midwives. Service and sacrifice have long been fundamental to the culture of midwifery in the NHS (Kirkham, 1999) and midwives have always made sacrifices in order to provide a good service. The professional autonomy to judge when extra efforts are called for now seems lacking in a system which requires an impossible, constant level of maximum effort.

The general and the particular

The way midwifery is taught in universities and the way it is practised within the NHS both focus on the general. Research inevitably generalizes and research-based guidelines apply to categories of clients, further encouraging us to fit those in our care into categories: high risk, teenagers and the obese are examples. Organizational pressures also encourage this categorization; for instance, 'latent phase of labour' is a useful category when the delivery suite is heaving but 'stay home and have a bath' may not be heard as helpful advice by an anxious woman in pain whose whole antenatal care has emphasized the importance of professional care in labour.

Such pressures to categorize discourage us from seeing women as individuals. Indeed those who do not accept their categorization are seen as disruptive and wasting valuable professional time. A less pleasant name for this approach is stereotyping (Kirkham *et al*, 2002).

Kindness is about individuals. An act is only experienced as kind if it meets the needs of the person to whom it is addressed. Generalizations as to being kind tend not to work. This is demonstrated whenever well trained shop assistants tell would-be customer to 'have a nice day' immediately after explaining to them that what they have requested cannot be supplied.

How can staff be kind when kindness is not valued by the organization?

Research has shown how individuals attempt to meet their professional ideals within the pressures of bureaucracy (Lipsky 1980). One way to do this is to provide excellent care to occasional clients who are seen as trustworthy. Such actions make professionals feel better, yet they are really an extreme form of stereotyping.

In healthcare in general, as well as maternity care in particular, dealing with patients within a highly fragmented service is easier and quicker to manage when staff do not engage with them as individuals. In her widely cited study of staff behaviour under these conditions, Isobel Menzies Lythe (1988) saw this response as a defence against anxiety. Yet it is a destructive coping strategy, for it is also a defence against the relationships which make kindness possible and against the job satisfaction which these relationships bring (Kirkham *et al*, 2006).

Midwives leave because their working context prevents them from giving high-quality care (Ball *et al*, 2002). Many move to alternative areas of work where they are better able to exercise kindness and compassion, and where the need for time to care is acknowledged, such as in hospice work.

Most NHS midwives work part-time. Some do so in order to have enough off duty time to recover from the demands of the job and to have the leeway to go beyond the call of duty when working (Kirkham *et al*, 2006). Many, if not most, NHS midwives regularly work beyond their contracted hours. Thus, those staff with the highest motivation, are taking less pay in order to work well. In so doing they are both collaborating with and subsidizing a system which is unkind to them and to their clients. They therefore struggle to care and to cope within a system which does not share their professional values and which exploits their commitment to those values.

Changing towards a kinder, relationship-based service

Birth is about relationships. It is important that midwife-mother relationships extend long enough for trust to be established and for kindness to be exercised and followed through. Continuity of care is therefore crucial. Ongoing relationships are rewarding for all concerned and especially valuable after stillbirth or other losses, when nurturing is all important (Kenworthy and Kirkham, 2009).

Continuity of care reduces the number of caring or colleague relationships to a human level. Such continuity can be achieved within a large modern maternity unit. The story of how this was done in St Georges Hospital, Sydney, Australia, is instructive and inspiring (Brodie and Homer, 2009). There is also detailed published guidance as to how such a transformation can be achieved (Homer *et al,* 2001 and 2008).

Though it has been UK Department of Health policy since 1993 (Department of Health, 1993), continuity of care is rare in the NHS. Caseloading projects and the relative autonomy of their midwives have often been seen as deviant within the current NHS management model and excellent schemes have been closed despite their good outcomes (Kirkham 2010). Midwives still struggle to make continuity of care available within the NHS and it can work very well: for example, a team 'providing caseload model of care to women with complex social risk factors' won the 2014 Royal College of Midwives Award (Midwives, 2014).

Models of continuity of midwifery care outside the NHS show what is possible, and efforts to contract these kinds of services into the NHS and into other maternity care systems around the world also deserve strong support. Nevertheless, it is politically naïve to ignore the vulnerability of such small services in the face of the massive commercial interests contracting into the modern NHS, and this is exacerbated in maternity care settings where private providers predominate.

A political context is needed for efforts towards relationship-based care to work. Midwives alone cannot achieve this. A strategic alliance of midwives, and mothers could work towards maternity care based on very different values. This would not be easy since the commercial values on which the NHS is based and the commodification of services runs right across our society. However, the recent NICE guidelines on intrapartum Care, that prioritize the support of maternity care systems that are likely to maximize good relationships, provide hope that change may be at hand (NICE, 2014).

Being kind to ourselves and our colleagues

As well as changing the service, we need to work upon our own skills. The short-term coping techniques, which many healthcare providers use to get through the work, damage us in the long run. Nor will such habits help us in a better future. Treating ourselves and our colleagues with kindness helps us and provides a role model for compassion. Caring for ourselves and our capacity to care help us towards working as we would wish to work. There are a number of actions we can take to achieve this end, and these are summarized in the key action points below.

Support from colleagues and others is crucial, and it is important to consciously set up a network of positive support as part of everyday professional life, and not just in a crisis. This should include colleagues we can talk to without fear of blame, someone we can ring when things have gone wrong, and someone who will listen and help us to understand and learn from our experiences. Colleagues, friends, and service users could be involved. Independent midwives offer a good model for such support networks.

Praise where it is due warms colleague relationships. Senior midwives and obstetricians may experience little praise, so when it is given it is remembered. Praise deserved can lessen feelings of professional isolation and mistrust. Beyond this, awareness of good practice should lead us to praise ourselves when appropriate and thus sustain our practice. Praise could be built into practice, as a counterbalance to blame. Regular meetings to analyze, praise and learn from good practice could teach more than the perinatal mortality meetings that are dreaded by many staff given the current maternity care context where they are afflicted with guilt and accustomed to blame.

Self-awareness is vital if our practice is to be both kind and resilient and we are not to be stretched beyond our sustainable limits. The necessary insight into our practice and behaviour can only be developed where we feel safe. Private writing can offer reflection with safety as 'reflective practice' (Bolton, 2001), or creative writing (1999) using notebooks or blogs or similar techniques. Journal writing can be painful in its honesty as well as self-affirming (Johns, 2004). Writing is a good way to detach ourselves slightly from our experience in order to examine it without being bowled over by the associated emotions, then we can decide what we can learn from the experience. Meditation can serve the same purpose, as can the various techniques of mindfulness. A degree of detachment is essential if we are to step back from our experience sufficiently to examine it, to understand our own needs as well as those of our clients and to see how we could do better. This is utterly different from professional dissociation (Garratt, 2010) which keeps us emotionally separate from an experience that is too painful to handle and which serves to hide that experience and cut us off from others and from mutual help. Skills of detachment and reflection can be developed in groups, based on ground rules which enable members to feel safe. Group reflection brings the potential for personal support and cross-fertilization of ideas.

Communications skills can be developed to achieve a degree of openness beyond the 'defensive routines' that currently protect us and the flaws of our current system. Some achieve this through 'nonviolent communication' (Rosenberg, 2003): a technique for focusing compassionately structured attention to the observations, feelings, needs and requests of both parties in an interaction. This structuring of response enables practitioners to cut through defensive habits that limit the degree to which we attend to ourselves and to others. Some practitioners draw techniques for achieving open communication from religious traditions. For example, Johns (2004) uses Buddhist techniques of mindfulness to focus his attention on his clients in palliative care. Another way of approaching this is through 'dialogue', an approach aimed at uncovering the common meaning in a group or an individual. The starting point for dialogue is always listening (Dixon, 1998), as it should be for midwifery in particular, and maternity care in general. Kindness is grounded in listening.

All of these techniques require us to honour ourselves as well as others. Jenny Patterson's Capacitar workshops have helped many midwives (knotstressed.com) and offer different ways in which we can increase our personal and professional resources. Honouring the kinds of skills which tend to be discounted in the modern NHS can also make us more aware and more committed to change. Embodied knowledge is one important example (Williams, 2014). While it may not be valued, it plays a large part in the wisdom of midwives and of mothers. Active Hope (Macy and Johnson, 2012) is another useful practice, which opens up hopeful ways of being.

The practice of all of the skills and techniques outlined in this section can change us. The response of others to the exercise of these approaches can be mutually inspiring. Such practices require a safe setting, some degree of skill and hope that things can change, if they are to be sustained (Dixon, 1998) and are easiest to develop in settings where there is a degree of professional autonomy.

Conclusions: Towards the future

Midwives are capable of giving truly compassionate care, where mothers are treated as adults. Such kindness nurtures all concerned. It takes time and requires a flexible work situation where the midwife has autonomy as to how her time is best used. Organizational change is needed for such time to be seen as well spent. Midwives cannot achieve this alone, but in alliance with service users and with other maternity professional colleagues, real change could be achieved.

Meanwhile it helps for all maternity care providers to work on their own skills and self awareness. This is not so as to prop up a system the basic values of which we do not share. We all need to do this for our own sanity, the job satisfaction that comes from good relationships with mothers, and because well supported childbearing women become strong mothers. Any lesser approach to kindness sees good midwives in particular as simply polite technicians, processing clients with a smile; a development of the obedient technicians described by Ruth Deery (2008). We, and the colleagues we work with in all the maternity care professions, can be so much more than that.

KEY MESSAGES

- Maternity care in the UK NHS and in many other settings around the world takes place in healthcare systems that are increasingly commercialized, commodified, and framed by risk-averse bureaucracies.
- These health system characteristics limit the potential for staff and service users to form the positive relationships that are the core of optimal maternity care.
- It is not enough to require practitioners working in maternity care to be kind and compassionate without addressing these toxic drivers.
- To mitigate at least some of the adverse effects of working in such environments, midwives and other maternity care staff need to develop supportive tools and techniques, including social support networks.

ACTION POINTS

- Set up your personal support system.
- Give praise where it is due.
- Develop self-awareness skills – seek out tools and techniques for doing this.
- Learn and practise open communication skills.
- Recognize that many of the skills you have are essential for high-quality care of women and babies and honour your expertise in these areas.

17 Caring for ourselves: the key to resilience

Billie Hunter and Lucie Warren

Jane and Kathy are experienced midwives currently working on the labour ward of a busy obstetric-led unit. Jane is concerned as Kathy seems upset. She's aware that Kathy had a very difficult shift the day before, looking after a woman whose care became complicated and eventually resulted in an emergency caesarean section. Kathy tells Jane that she was so upset by what happened that she burst into tears as soon as she got into her car to go home. To help her relax, Kathy drank a couple of glasses of wine before bed, but wasn't able to switch off and slept badly. She was anxious about coming back to the unit this afternoon. These days she is 'just waiting for something bad to happen' in work. She says 'I'm not like you – you always seem confident and enjoy your job'. Jane tries to reassure Kathy and tells her that all midwives have difficult days. A couple of months ago Jane had a similarly difficult situation, and had felt much better after meeting up with a colleague for a coffee outside of work and talking through what had happened. It helped her get things into perspective and reminded her of all the good things about being a midwife.

The vignette above highlights the very real pressure midwives can feel. But we can spot some differences here. Kathy is struggling to cope, whilst Jane appears to be managing well and finds work rewarding. She could be said to demonstrate professional 'resilience'.

What is resilience?

Resilience is a term that is gaining popularity in contemporary media and has its roots in psychology. It has been defined as a positive individual, community or societal response to adverse circumstances (e.g. environmental disasters, political upheaval, personal trauma or economic adversity). Personal characteristics such as being optimistic can aid individuals in responding positively to adversity (Jacelon, 1997), but there is also evidence that resilience can be a 'learned process' where coping mechanisms are developed over time (Ungar, 2012). Much of the work around resilience has focused on assisting children, young people and families to adapt to emotional/physical/psychological challenges, social disadvantage and inequality (Hart, Blincow and Thomas, 2007). Professional resilience is an area which is less well explored.

Midwives are known to be especially vulnerable to stress and burnout as frequent emotional demands, often unrecognized, are a crucial aspect of the job (Hunter, 2006). Exploring and identifying effective ways of coping and thriving within the workplace could benefit midwives in achieving a long and rewarding career.

So what do we know about professional resilience in the caring professions? A small number of studies have explored resilience in public service work (e.g. nursing, social work, psychology, counselling and medicine) and identified individual factors that appear to support resilient responses such as optimism, self-awareness, and self-efficacy (McCann *et al*, 2013). Several other factors also appear to help professionals actively manage and cope with adversity. These tend to be proactive behaviours such as managing a good work/life balance, being reflective and accessing peer support or mentoring (Hodges, Keeley and Troyan, 2008; Jackson *et al*, 2011; McAllister and Mckinnon, 2009). However it is unclear whether these findings can be applied to midwifery. Midwives like Jane may provide insights into how some practitioners are able to be resilient, cope well and thrive in maternity care, despite difficult circumstances.

Research into midwifery resilience

In our research study (Hunter and Warren, 2013, 2014) we asked experienced clinical midwives like Jane to tell us how they thought they had become resilient. Was this a personal trait or something they had developed? Did they differ from their colleagues and how? What factors helped or hindered resilience?

This is the first study to focus specifically on midwifery resilience, so we used a qualitative approach to 'test the water' and explore whether the idea of resilience held any meaning for midwives and, if so, what that meaning was. Eleven midwives who described themselves as being able to 'bounce back after a difficult day' took part in a month-long online discussion group. We analyzed these conversations looking for common themes (for further details of the study's design and findings, see Hunter and Warren, 2013, 2014).

Three key approaches to being resilient were identified:

1. Reactive strategies: day-to-day managing and coping. Practical coping strategies, developed over time, were used to get a short-term sense of perspective on work adversities. These included:
   - reflection (either alone or with trusted colleagues)
   - using positive mood changers such as music and exercise
   - accessing social support
   - attempting to keep a good work-life balance.
   In short – the midwives tried to control whatever was possible in

their lives and accept what they had no control over.

2. Developing self-awareness: self-awareness and 'knowing yourself' was seen as important. This included an element of self-protection, looking after yourself by having realistic self-expectations and managing the expectations of others. The midwives described how a strong professional identity and love of midwifery practice contributed to this core sense of who they were. There was a moral dimension to this: feeling that you are 'making a difference' and contributing to the greater good was important for keeping a sense of balance.

3. Proactive strategies: Building resilience in yourself and others. The midwives thought that it was possible to develop personal resilience over time, and also to support others to build their resilience. Ways of doing this included proactively learning techniques for self-protection (such as increasing self-awareness of potential triggers), and supporting and empowering others (especially less experienced colleagues). Critical moments were noted when midwives were most susceptible to adversity and would need most support: when newly qualified and after a difficult clinical experience.

These key approaches are illustrated below. In the table on the next page we provide a Resilient Repertoire, linked to the model and developed from the findings of our research. We suggest that you could use this repertoire as a helpful 'toolkit' for caring for yourself and developing professional resilience.

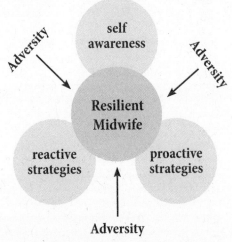

Figure 1: Model of Midwifery Resilience

Table: Resilient Repertoire

MANAGING & COPING (reactive)

Gain perspective	Gain a sense of perspective through the use of reflection either on your own or with colleagues. Reflection can help to make sense of a situation.
Social support	Social support is key to resilience. Access support from friends or trusted colleagues. Talk to them about how you feel.
Mood changers	Use strategies to improve mood. These could be calming such as music or warm baths that help you to unwind or slightly more stimulating activities like walking the dog or exercising.
Work-life balance	Develop a fulfilling personal life with outside interests and try to keep work and home life separate.
Self-efficacy	Understand and acknowledge strengths and abilities. A sense of belief in your capability builds confidence.

SELF-AWARENESS

Autonomy	Where possible take control of those aspects of work that you are able to whilst accepting that there are some elements outside of your control.
Identity	A strong professional identity and love of midwifery practice can sustain you through difficult times. Recognize and value the difference you and your profession can make to the women and families you care for.
Obligation to oneself	Look after your own needs. Be aware of your capabilities and limitations and avoid unreasonable self-expectations and manage the expectations of others.

BUILDING RESILIENCE (proactive)

Protective self-management	Anticipate stress and recognize the warning signs in yourself and others. Take active steps to manage or avoid challenging situations or hindering relationships.
Support colleagues	Identify and support those colleagues who may feel vulnerable such as student and newly qualified midwives or those who have been affected by a difficult or emotionally challenging case. This encourages and promotes a caring and supportive work environment.
Learning and investment	Resilience can be a learnt process and it is possible to find strength in adversity. Learn what worked for you and others in previous challenging experiences and adapt these ways of coping to new challenges.
Facilitate empowerment	Nurture and encourage colleagues; recognize and acknowledge when they have done well. It is important to promote and protect optimism in yourself and others to create a positive working environment.

Conclusion

Midwives frequently report feeling under pressure and burnt out for many reasons, that may affect the way they deliver care. However, some midwives appear to be resilient to the stresses they face. Our study suggests resilience can be learned and developed over time. Whilst we have suggested strategies for self-awareness and building resilience, we stress the importance of combining resilience with compassion and respect, for yourself, your work colleagues, and the women you care for.

KEY MESSAGES

- Evidence tells us that not all midwives are coping. Low morale, stress and burnout are reported and may affect the quality of compassionate care.
- But some midwives do cope – i.e. they are resilient in the face of workplace adversity. Research evidence suggests that resilience is not just a character trait but can be learnt and developed over time.
- A Model of Midwifery Resilience and a Resilient Repertoire, developed in discussion with experienced midwives, offers some insights. The Repertoire includes short-term and long-term strategies for day-to-day coping, developing self-awareness, and building resilience in yourself and others.
- Using the Repertoire may be a helpful framework for looking after yourself and developing resilience.
- Caution! Resilience must not be seen as becoming hard/distant/toughened up. Resilience needs to be combined with compassion and respect – for yourself, your colleagues and the families you serve.

ACTION POINTS

- If you have had a difficult shift/case, talk it over with friends or colleagues to get some perspective. And offer them the same support in return.
- Make time to do something you enjoy that will help you to feel good. It can be as simple as going for a walk.
- Be aware of those colleagues around you who may be struggling; empathy and encouragement can help to make it easier.
- Notice how you feel when you are stressed and what situations make you feel stressed. Manage self-expectations and those of others!
- Remember the value of the wonderful work you do. You really can make a difference.

PART III

MAKING IT HAPPEN:
SOLUTIONS FROM AROUND THE WORLD

18 Clinical guidelines: hindrance or help for respectful compassionate care?

Julie Frohlich and Rineke Schram

In the majority of countries throughout the world, decisions around the design of maternity services are in the hands of policy makers and, to a lesser degree, of maternity care workers. Expectant mothers, and indeed parents, seem to be passive recipients in the main. Even though in the United Kingdom health policy is increasingly instructing healthcare workers to support shared decision making (SDM) processes, with the patient at the centre (DH, 2012; DH, 2013), there is a disconnect between these policies, and what happens in reality.

Use of the words 'allowed' and 'not allowed' in the context of maternity care illustrates the point. When there is a misunderstanding of the meaning of the words 'clinical guideline' and the use of them, maternity care workers can be afraid to support women's choices. This in turn may lead to dehumanized disrespectful care, with compliance with guidance taking priority. This chapter, written by a midwife and an obstetrician, explores these issues from a multidisciplinary perspective, using guidelines as a starting point, and suggests ways in which maternity care can move forward in the coming decade to bring to fruition the care choice promises of the past.

What is a guideline?

There appears to be a great deal of confusion amongst midwives and doctors about the precise definition and role of clinical guidelines. Our observation is that the words 'guidelines', 'policies' and 'protocols' are often used interchangeably. This is both wrong and potentially damaging to the cause of individualized care. The UK National Collaborating Centre for Women's and Children's Health (NCCWCH) state that a guideline is: 'A systematically developed tool that describes aspects of a patient's condition and the care to be given. A good guideline makes recommendations about treatment and care based on the best research available, rather than opinion. It is used to assist clinician and patient decision making about appropriate health care for specific clinical conditions.' (NCCWCH, 2007:xiv)

It is interesting that the emphasis here is on 'recommendations' because a recommendation is something that can be accepted or declined. Except in exceptional circumstances, when it is considered that a patient lacks the competence to make their own decision, there can be no enforced adherence to a particular recommendation. The competent patient is always free to choose. The phrase '*Assist clinician and patient decision making*' is also important as it implies discussion, sharing and mutual agreement as to a planned course of treatment or care. In the words of the Chairman of NICE, Professor David Haslam (Responsible Officer's Conference Brighton, June 2014), '*Guidelines are not tramlines – use with, not at patients*'.

In contrast, a policy is a way of doing something that has been officially agreed by an organization. A policy is non-negotiable. Every UK Trust has a whole raft of human relations (HR) policies that apply equally and without deviation to all its employees. This lack of deviation is designed to ensure clarity and equality. For example, if a midwife or doctor turns up to work in a clinical area wearing strappy high-heeled sandals, shorts and a low-cut vest top, stating her intention to wear these items for the duration of her shift, she is likely to be in breach of her employer's uniform policy and could be disciplined accordingly. In effect, the uniform policy obligates the midwife or doctor to conform – it is not a matter of choice.

Finally, a protocol is an agreed and written method for carrying out a specific procedure, a scientific experiment or a course of medical treatment within an organization. A protocol is task related and tends to focus on one specific area. For example, there could be a protocol for changing a surgical dressing following a caesarean section. Like policies, the emphasis here is on compliance; a protocol is not a decision-making tool, rather it is an 'ABC' of how to carry out a specific procedure.

From the brief explanations offered above it is clear that guidelines, policies and protocols have distinct and differing roles within an organization. All have their place, but they are not, and never should be, viewed as interchangeable. Until we appreciate these differing definitions, and in particular the precise and unique role of guidelines in informing clinical decision making, we will never be able to use them to their best advantage, for the benefit of the women who use maternity services.

The potential benefits and disbenefits of guidelines

When a guideline is written and used well, it has the potential both to raise standards of care and to reduce variation in the availability and provision of care; it can offer a 'gold standard' for benchmarking. Guidelines can bring together the appraisal and assimilation of the best available quantitative and qualitative research evidence and consolidate expert opinion so that they can be used to inform clinical decision making in partnership with women and discourage interventions of no proven benefit. Guidelines should be clear about their scope and explicit about what is and isn't known about a subject. They should be concise and easy to read and access. Guidelines have the potential to improve outcomes and to improve safety.

However, there are also several potential pitfalls associated with guidelines. When written and used badly, there can be an over-emphasis on 'hard evidence' that encourages a dictatorial, 'standard' approach to care, restricting rather than facilitating choice. There can be a tendency to focus on specific and immediate, short-term outcomes promoting a medicalized approach to care, rather than considering longer-term outcomes and overall well-being. Most worryingly, guidelines can be applied punitively, both for the practitioner whose care strays outside of the guideline and for the woman who dares to ask for something different. In the words of Sheila Kitzinger:

> *When a woman is admitted to hospital she encounters a social system that regulates her behaviour and that of everyone else in it. There is a bureaucracy designed to ensure conformity and obedience and a hierarchical management structure that punishes deviance and rewards uncritical adherence to the rules and protocols it dictates.* (Kitzinger, 2006:17)

So, at their best, guidelines can be an effective decision-making tool, but at their worst they are restricting for all parties.

Evidence-based medicine

In 1996, David Sackett, professor of evidence-based medicine (EBM) at Oxford, and several other academics published an editorial in the *BMJ* (Sackett *et al*, 1996). This editorial has been widely quoted as it provides a considered consensus of what EBM is, and perhaps more importantly, what it is not. The authors stated that evidence-based medicine is: '...*the conscientious, explicit and judicious use of current best evidence in making decisions about the care of individual patients*'. And that '*Good doctors* [and midwives] *use both individual clinical expertise and the best available external evidence, and neither alone is enough*'. The authors went on to explain that evidence-based medicine is not '..."*cook book" medicine*', '...*cost-cutting medicine*' or '...*restricted to randomised trials and meta-analysis*'.

In effect, the authors acknowledged that external clinical research evidence can inform, but can never replace individual clinical expertise, or patients' values. In consultation with the service user, it is this expertise and these values that decide whether or not the external evidence applies on a case by case basis and, if so, how it should best be integrated into a clinical decision.

The editorial warns against the dangers of a 'guideline culture' dictating standardized care: '*Without clinical expertise, practice risks becoming tyrannised by evidence, for even excellent external evidence may be inapplicable to or inappropriate for an individual patient*.' Tyrannized is a strong word and there is much in this editorial to celebrate as it absolutely endorses individualized care. More recently, Greenhalgh *et al* (2014) advocate a return to 'true' EBM: individualized for the patient, using judgement, not rules.

Midwives and obstetricians who find themselves challenged by senior managers about care decisions 'outside the guidelines' may be advised to cite the above publications, and in particular the highly regarded editorial from Sackett *et al* (1996), in defending their rationale for facilitating individualized care.

The law in relation to the choice agenda

Difficulties with the principle of informed choice occur when either the practitioner perceives that there is a 'right choice' to be made on the part of the woman (usually in keeping with a guideline) or when the woman's perceived 'right choice' for herself is in conflict with the knowledge, beliefs and/or experience of the clinician or with guideline recommendations.

In such circumstances it is understandably tempting for the clinician to attempt to 'steer' the woman towards their own recommendations for care, especially when there are perceived safety concerns. There can be no doubt that most clinicians believe they have the woman's and the baby's best interests at heart. However, our duty of care cannot ever justify the coercion and bullying tactics many of us, midwives and obstetricians, have witnessed and/or employed over the years. Whatever the motivation, we make a mockery of 'counselling' and 'informed choice' when only partial information is given and crucial counterbalancing information is withheld; this is especially so when information is given in an emotionally charged or 'loaded' way.

Under UK common law, minimum acceptable standards of clinical care derive from responsible customary practice, not from guidelines (Hurwitz, 1999). That is not to say that guidelines do not provide courts with a benchmark for clinical care, but it has also been argued that to implement faulty guidelines, or recommendations from guidelines without appropriate informed consent, could in itself be interpreted as negligent (Hurwitz, 2004).

The charitable organization Birthrights provides a comprehensive summary of women's rights and we would urge every midwife and obstetrician to spend some time navigating its website (www.birthrights. org.uk). Birthrights states that 'Pregnant women are entitled to make autonomous decisions in the same way as any other person, and their decisions must be respected, regardless of whether health professionals agree with them'. Birthrights goes on to explain that health professionals have a duty to explain the risks and benefits of any procedure or care option (including for the unborn child) but they must not apply 'undue pressure' to 'encourage' the woman to make a particular choice. The law then is on the side of the woman as far as making informed choices about her own care is concerned. Elizabeth Prochaska, lawyer and founder of Birthrights, has elaborated on human rights and childbirth in Chapter 3.

Using risk perceptions to limit choice

Many women over the years have experienced the 'not allowed' philosophy along the lines of 'Of course, what I really wanted was… a home birth/to use the pool during labour/to have my baby on the MLU (Maternity and Labour Unit)/not to have continuous monitoring…' (the list is endless) 'but the doctor/midwife said I was not allowed'. This authoritarian approach may contribute to the perception of unkindness, or lack of respect and has the potential to initiate a feeling of powerlessness.

The rationale for denial of choice often sounds plausible enough 'because of my age', 'because I had some heavy bleeding last time' (ironically, often attributable to unnecessary obstetric intervention), because I am 'high risk' and, increasingly in recent years, 'because of my BMI'. Sadly, the reality is that all too often clinicians are simply trying to justify a 'one size fits all' approach to maternity care and the rationale for this stance is adherence to a clinical guideline. We do not facilitate women's 'informed choice' because of some minor deviation from being completely 'low risk'. Instead, we navigate women towards 'informed compliance' with whatever is recommended in the relevant guideline.

Informed choice and informed compliance are fundamentally different concepts. Informed choice relies on honesty, respect and mutual trust; no information is withheld and information sharing is done impartially and with no hidden agenda for either party; effective communication is key. Informed choice leads ultimately to 'informed consent', to an agreed treatment, intervention or course of action and nobody can give meaningful informed consent without the counter option of informed refusal: the two go together.

In our experience, women who request care 'outside guidelines' have often had a previous highly medicalized labour and birth culminating in operative or instrumental delivery. Women report having experienced feelings of complete lack of control without the ability (or option) to make ongoing informed choices about their care. They recall feeling both vulnerable and frightened. Often it appears that women have little time to reflect as they are swept along by the busyness of new motherhood, and they tend to compartmentalize these previous 'bad' labour and birth experiences. However, it appears that the traumatizing events of labour surface with acute clarity when the woman is pregnant again and she knows with absolute certainty that she cannot and will not be subject to that same lack of control ever again.

The importance of flexibility in response to the unexpected

One of the biggest dangers of a documented, individualized care plan, especially if it has been difficult to navigate, is a tendency to see it as somehow 'final' and inflexible. This is especially so if it has been discussed and agreed with a senior clinician, as junior staff may be wary of amending it later on for fear of offending. When facilitating individual informed choices, we must ensure that everyone involved understands that any agreed care plan is just that — it is a plan and not a contract to be adhered to come what may. The essence of every good care plan is that both parties (the woman and the clinicians) understand that the agreed plan is not 'set in stone'. If circumstances change at whatever stage of the pregnancy continuum then the plan should be revisited, the new circumstances discussed and a revised plan should be agreed and documented.

In essence, the process of effective care planning is iterative. The consequences of not understanding this necessary flexibility could be dire. No clinician, no matter how senior, has the ability to see into the future. To stick to an original plan in such circumstances could jeopardize the safety of the woman and her baby.

Linked to this issue is the question of support (or lack of support) for the midwife or obstetrician who facilitates a woman's informed choice outside a local clinical guideline and his/her fear of retribution if s/he does. Every midwife and doctor has contractual obligations to his/her employer, and his/her contract may even specify that s/he should offer care that is consistent with the agreed clinical guidelines in place at that Trust.

However, in the UK the registered midwife also has professional obligations outlined in the NMC Code (NMC, 2008) and the Midwives rules and standards (NMC, 2012). These include that midwives '...must treat people as individuals and respect their dignity' and '…must respect and support people's rights to accept or decline treatment and care'.

Doctors have responsibilities under the GMC's Good Medical Practice – The duties of a doctor registered with the General Medical Council code of conduct (2013) that require a doctor to 'Work in partnership with patients, listen to, and respond to, their concerns and preferences, give patients the information they want or need in a way they can understand and respect patients' right to reach decisions with you about their treatment and care.' And finally, 'to support patients in caring for themselves to improve and maintain their health.' The GMC's supplementary guidance on consent further clarifies: 'You should give information to patients in a balanced way. If you recommend a particular treatment or course of action, you should explain your reasons for doing so. But you must not put pressure on a patient to accept your advice.' and 'You must give information about risk in a balanced way. You should avoid bias, and you should explain the expected benefits as well as the potential burdens and risks of any proposed investigation or treatment.' (GMC, 2008)

In essence, then, every NHS midwife and doctor has a duty to inform the woman about the evidence and advice contained within national and local guidelines and even to offer clear recommendations for care in line with those guidelines. But a midwife or doctor would be in breach of his/her professional obligations if s/he attempted to enforce a treatment or procedure that the woman declines, even if it is recommended in a guideline.

Conclusion

If we could remove one word from our midwifery and obstetric dialogue with women it should be the word 'allow'. There is not, nor ever can there be, a 'one size fits all' approach to maternity care. If, in our attempts to 'standardize' care through the rigid adherence to guidelines and to 'eliminate' risk, we view women simply as physical beings or vessels for the developing fetus, we fail to understand the uniqueness of what it is to be human.

Uncomfortable as it undoubtedly sometimes is, if we are really to embrace the concept of women's individual informed choices we have to mature as practitioners. We have to move away from a paternalistic 'the doctor (or midwife) knows best' model and embrace instead the concepts of women's autonomy and partnership working. We have to learn to trust women to make educated choices about their own care, even if this occasionally involves women making 'wrong' choices from our own perspective. We can know the guidelines inside out; what we can never know to the same extent is what makes each woman under our care unique. In the novel *The Unlikely Pilgrimage of Harold Fry*, the eponymous Mr Fry comes to the realization that '...*everyone was the same, and also unique; and that this was the dilemma of being human*' (Joyce, 2012: 181). This, in a nutshell, is what we as practitioners have similarly to understand.

It is clear from countless anecdotal accounts from midwives and obstetricians, and from women's own experiences, that it is possible to facilitate women's individual choices safely and sustainably within mainstream maternity services. With the support of policy makers who have already endorsed this approach, our challenge now is to ensure that every woman has the same opportunity to exercise her right to individual, informed choice and that we put an end to the 'postcode lottery' of care still currently on offer within NHS maternity services. The consequences of not embracing this challenge proactively and constructively are really too depressing to contemplate

KEY MESSAGES

- Guidelines must be based on independent high-quality evidence that is both practicable, robust and can be individualized.
- If this is achieved, guidelines can raise standards, increase compassionate maternity care, and reduce variation in the availability and provision of care.
- Guidelines provide guidance and recommendations, they must never be used to dictate care.
- Guidelines must not hinder the practice and application of clinical expertise and shared decision making, and of respectful attitudes and behaviours.

ACTION POINTS

- Use guidelines to facilitate shared decision making and individualized care.
- Understand the evidence that guidelines are based upon, and whether there are weaknesses in that evidence, e.g. value judgements.
- Consider how you communicate 'risk' and whether that promotes knowledge, understanding, and respectful compassionate care.
- Challenge the use of the word 'allow' when discussing management or care plans.

This chapter is based on an original article: Frohlich J. *MIDIRS Midwifery Digest* 2013;23(3):279-287.

19 Making it happen in China

Ngai Fen Cheung

With a population of over 130 million, China is becoming the world's largest economy, undergoing tremendous social developments while continuing strict implementation of a single child birth-control policy. China is on track to achieve the Millennium Development Goals 4 and 5 for maternal/ infant health. However, this success has come at some cost, especially in terms of increasing interventions in childbirth, and a decreasing emphasis on compassionate care. Very recently, moves towards increasing midwife-led normal birth units (MNBU) in China have, anecdotally, brought care and compassion back into maternity care, resulting in an increased sense of wellbeing for both childbearing women, and attending staff.

This chapter explores the potential consequences of the loss of a midwifery sensibility in maternity care in China, and one particular initiative to try to reverse this process.

The nature of maternity care in China

Antenatal and postnatal care in China is mainly composed of routine medical check-ups, scans, and tests with very little personal interaction. Care is highly clinically focused, with little regard for the needs and views of women and their families. In terms of intrapartum care, there is evidence of extreme variation. For example, maternity hospitals in developed urban regions of the country have caesarean section rates (CSR) ranging between 46% and 100% (Huang, 2000, WHO, 2010) while caesarean section rates are lower than 10% in some low-income regions. The average rate is over 36% across the country as a whole (UNICEF, 2012). In particular, caesarean section with no medical indication is over 40% (Pang, 2010), the highest in the world (WHO, 2010a, b).

Some of this highly technocratic systems-led care is due to routine hospitalization and expensive technical 'quick-fixes', which are taking the place of woman-centred approaches based on supporting the normal physiology of labour and birth. Overtreatment has been rising in China since the 1990s, and midwifery has been increasingly marginalized. As both of these changes have gathered pace, there has been less and less emphasis on some of the fundamental aspects of maternity care, including compassion (DoH, 2012), ethical obligations, and respect for individuals, both women and midwives.

Finding a solution: setting up midwife-led normal birth units in China

Around ten years ago, the high iatrogenic CSRs in China started to raise alarm bells among a small group of Chinese midwives, and overseas collaborators. This led to an exploratory study on CS decision making (CDM) in China which was supported by a Sino-British Fellowship from the British Academy and a Small Project Fund from the University of Edinburgh. The project ran between 2004 and 2006. The main findings of the CDM study were: the demise of midwifery; over-reliance on obstetricians and technologies; and the absence of evidence-based research information for informed choices (Cheung *et al*, 2005a,b, 2006a,b).

Informed by the above findings, the first MNBU was designed and set up in China. After two years of preparation, the Unit was eventually established in Hangzhou in 2008 with 'two-to-one' intrapartum supportive care (midwife, birth companion and woman), and face-to-face, virtual (communications and consultations) and tele-midwifery care (eg, video-classes, video-monitoring and inquiries). In contrast to the very high levels of caesarean section in the surrounding hospitals, the vaginal birth rate in the unit was 87.6% in the first six months and it has remained at 90-94% ever since.

Midwives based in the MNBU have taken pride from their 24/7 service, and in its safety record, and women's highly positive accounts of their experiences (Cheung, 2009; Cheung *et al*, 2009, 2011a,b,c; Mander *et al*, 2009). This has also heightened their own sense of self-esteem, as confirmed by a story told by one of the midwives working in the MNBU:

> *I have been a midwife for over thirty years. When I just started this job, I had the instinct to provide the compassionate care to women, but my efforts were swamped by the existing busy maternity system. I'm glad that I have eventually learned through working in this Midwife-led unit. It helps me to understand and confirm eventually what midwifery is and how a midwife should work. I'm also glad to be able to understand, finally, after these years, at the nearly end of my career, that safe supportive care during childbirth is essential for a midwife; indeed, it is the essence of midwifery.*

Rolling out the benefits

The political leaders in the city where the MNBU was set up very soon realized the benefits of the kind of care provided there, and decreed that all midwives working in other institutions in the city should undertake a rotation to the unit for three months to enable them to learn how to support normal birth (Downe, 2011). They realized that the model demonstrated the link between effective, compassionate midwifery care and normality in terms of labour and birth (Pan and Cheung, 2011).

The demand for the MNBU services is increasing, and other areas around the country are beginning to work towards setting up such services locally. The following story of a second-time mother expresses this view:

> *I had a lovely normal birth in this unit. It is great to have my husband and the midwife with me throughout the labour. That was very reassuring. They always offered me a cup of drinks, a relaxing massage and made a little chat. When my birth was getting difficult, the midwife stayed very cool and kept on explaining, encouraging and reassuring me and my husband. The rapport developed during the antenatal care and the labour allowed me to feel confident and to make it through the labour. The birth I had previously in my hometown helps me appreciate the care I had in this unit. I've never seen this kind of good service before. It is excellent! I hope this kind of wonderful service can be available everywhere in the country.*

Next steps

Based on the above experience and supported by the first ever newly established Chinese Midwifery Research Unit, midwives in the area took an active part in a related international EU project focused on maximizing salutogenic maternity care (EU COST Action IS0907) and in hosting the 7th International Normal Labour and Birth Research Conference in Hangzhou, China, in 2012. Through these interactions and exchanges, the first national Midwifery Expert Committee was established on 4th May 2013. The Committee and the midwife members pledged their engagement in calling for the government's political and legal commitment to address neglect. A way forward is in the process of being devised.

ICM Gap Analysis Workshop

It was against this background that a two-day International Confederation of Midwives (ICM) Gap Analysis Workshop took place from 26th to 27th March 2014 to look into issues of education, regulation and association of the development of midwifery in China. The participants were policy-makers, the Chinese Maternal and Child Health Association, the Chinese Nursing Association, the Society of Perinatal Medicine, the Chinese Medical Association, the Women's Association, Higher Educational

Institutions, the United Nations Population Fund, and non-governmental organizations in China.

Forty leaders in education, regulation and association were invited to attend the workshop but over 120 turned up. A joint call for action was reached by the end of the event, setting out the vision, mission, commitments and actions for midwifery development as a long-term strategy to improve the health and overall wellbeing of women, newborns and families

Why the new model works

The Chinese MNBU model works both practically and conceptually. Practically, the 'two-to-one' approach constitutes an effective social support for women and provides midwives with an independent working space. Conceptually, the MNBU practice is dependent on its belief about the normality of childbirth, and the importance of kindness, care, respect and compassion. This links physiological and social-cultural process, and does not supervalue the need to risk out all unforeseen pathological changes. This in turn raises questions about the prophylactic use of technological interventions in normal labour and birth. Through the ICM Gap Analysis Workshop, the status of Chinese midwives was given due recognition, as were the fundamental rights of women and newborns. A strategy for change, and an action research study, were designed with six fundamental values as underpinned by the British Department of Health: care, compassion, competence, communication, courage and commitment (DoH, 2012) to support professionals and care staff to deliver appropriate maternity care. Chinese midwives are now aware that they need to develop a national midwives association and build on their commitments to improve the care and experience of their clients to meet the changing needs of women, newborns, families and carers.

Conclusion

The MNBU practice challenges the technically orientated maternity care system in China. It highlights how kindness, compassion and respect matter in maternity care, and how they can be optimized in service design and in practice. The recent national and international research collaborations, including the ICM Gap Analysis, the COST Action IS0907 and the Normal Labour and Birth 7th International Research Conference held in Hangzhou, have already to a large extent encouraged midwifery practice there. These have initiated a favourable shift of emphasis. Maternity care is no longer concerned with safety alone. There is now a new focus on both safety and positive experiences. Midwives in China are beginning to be perceived nationally as an indispensable care workforce for maternal health; and kindness and compassion are being understood as being important to the country's healthcare reform alongside its rapid economic, social and technological progress.

KEY MESSAGES

- Midwives are the backbone of maternity services for the health and wellbeing of women, newborns and families.
- The Midwifery Normal Birth Unit model works in China.
- Kindness and compassion are essential components of maternity services in every country.

ACTION POINTS

- Governments need to promote midwifery as a profession nationally with appropriate policies, codes of conduct and terms of service.
- Midwifery research in education, regulation and association for the health and wellbeing of the general public needs to be supported by research funders and commissioners.
- Professional organizations and individual maternity care staff should consider using the ICM global standards as a guide to improve the quality of maternity services, and the capacity of staff to deliver good quality care.
- The rights of women, midwives, and all frontline staff should be mutually respected in maternity care design and delivery.

20 Making it happen in Brazil

Maria Helena Bastos

In the past 15 years in Brazil, nearly all children and women's health indicators, such as mortality and morbidity, as well as access to healthcare services, have improved (Victoria et al, 2011). Paradoxically, maternity care services are frequently considered unsafe, of poor quality, not based on the best evidence, with excessive use of harmful and inappropriate interventions, marked by an authoritarian provider-patient relationship, with underlying aspects related to discriminatory practices towards gender, social class and ethnicity (D'Orsi et al, 2014; Aguiar et al, 2013; Leal et al, 2005). There is a hospital-centred approach to healthcare in which pregnancy, labour and birth are seen as 'risky'. The removal of birth from its natural, safe and familiar environment and, more precisely, taking birth away from the control of women, have not contributed to improving health outcomes. The perception from the medical authorities is that a doctor's opinion is unquestionable and is 'best for the patient' permeates the imagery of the Brazilian healthcare system. Promoting evidence-based midwifery care is also a challenge.

The experience of childbirth is dominated by a climate of fear: fear of pain, fear of death, fear of what can happen to the mother or her baby, and the fear of being mistreated (McCallum and Reis, 2006). The fear imposed on women planning a normal birth is fed differently in both the public and private healthcare sectors. In the corridors of the SUS (the Brazilian public healthcare system) women say: 'you will be left suffering there for hours, until you have a vaginal birth'. In private hospitals doctors will try to convince women that caesarean section is less dangerous, more humane and less traumatic for the baby than normal birth. As a result, in the private sector over 88% of births are caesarean sections (Domingues et al, 2014).

Why does normal birth provoke such horror in both healthcare professionals and women? It is perhaps the result of obstetric training. There is also a sexual reproductive culture in Brazil which has a strong religious and misogynistic bias. Vaginal birth is seen as unbearable, dangerous, primitive, unpredictable, disgusting, dirty, shameful, and to be avoided whenever possible. Perhaps this explains why obsolete procedures such as routine episiotomy, use of drugs to accelerate delivery, such as synthetic oxytocin without safety protocols, manoeuvres on the uterus to force out the baby (ie, fundal pressure or Kristeller manoeuvre), in addition to immobilization of the woman in anti-physiologic positions (ie, lithotomy), and unnecessary caesarean sections remain standard practice.

The scenario we have today in Brazil is a culture which values medical procedures and the services provided by private healthcare, while trivializing the risks of interventions such as caesarean sections. The services provided by the public healthcare system and midwifery are undermined. As a result women have much less chance of receiving respectful and compassionate care and a normal birth

Institutional violence in obstetric care in Brazil

The birth of a child is an important event in the life of a woman. Unfortunately for some women birth is often remembered as a violent and traumatic experience in which the woman felt intimidated, disrespected and abused by those who should be providing healthcare. Despite the challenge and the complexity of this subject, humanization is a term widely accepted in Brazil as it is a less accusatory term than disrespect, abuse or violence. The Ministry of Health has adopted strategies to engage with healthcare providers about issues regarding institutional violence.

Research in Brazil reports on the dehumanization of reproductive healthcare, and the frequent abuse in the use of unnecessary, painful and even harmful interventions that are usually associated with higher morbidity and mortality to both mother and baby (Leal *et al,* 2014; Schraiber *et al,* 2009; D'Oliveira *et al,* 2002). According to Diniz (2005) the situations that might be considered 'dehumanizing' are: (a) the precarious working conditions that lead to failure, stress and psychological defence of healthcare professionals on the one hand, and long waiting times, poor access and poor reception of patients on the other; (b) the positivist approach of biomedical rationality that ignores the subjective, cultural and personal needs of patients, leading to an impersonal service provision, focused on risk management and illness and not the health and wellbeing; (c) the use of technology as a substitute for human relationships; and (d) the devaluation of communication and lack of empathy. Within this context, humanization is a process of transforming the culture and behaviour to acknowledge and respect users' and providers' subjective experiences, including sociocultural aspects, in order to improve working conditions and quality of care (Rattner, 2009).

Brazilian researchers consider institutional violence in obstetric care as the submission of women to unnecessary procedures and interventions that can result in a 'cascade of interventions', causing risk of harm to the health of the mother and/or the baby. Such unnecessary procedures and interventions in labour and birth include routine use of oxytocin for augmentation of labour contractions, denial of the right for companionship in birth, birthing in supine or lithotomy position, use of uterine fundal pressure to expedite delivery (ie, Kristeller manoeuvre), limited access to pain relief in labour, prophylactic use of forceps for academic training purposes and routine use of episiotomy.

In Brazil the concept of disrespect and abuse is mixed up with the concept of violence (Minayo, 2006). Nevertheless, we can identify some literature that tries to understand the determinants of institutional violence in obstetric care. In 2010 the Perseu Abramo Foundation conducted research on 'Brazilian women and gender in public and private spaces'. This survey identified that 25% of women reported some form of disrespect and abuse during care in labour and birth (eg, cursing, performing painful procedures without notice and/or consent, shouting, preventing the presence of a birth companion).

Institutional violence is trivialized by healthcare professionals through their use of a moral and discriminatory tone (joking comments such as 'you were not crying when you did it' or 'don't worry, next year you will be here again'). Threats are used as a way to persuade the patient, and the naturalization of labour pain is presented as the price to be paid to become a mother (Aguiar, 2013). The widespread institutional violence also points to the trivialization of injustice and the suffering of others as a social phenomenon that affects the whole of society, weakening the ties of personal interaction between professionals and patients. The crystallization of class stereotypes and gender are reflected in the care of these patients and contribute to the invisibility of violence as a theme for reflection and institutional control.

The term 'obstetric violence' has been described in several countries in Latin America. In Venezuela, Mexico and Argentina, obstetric violence is recognized as a crime against women and something which should be prevented, punished and eradicated. In Brazil obstetric violence is characterized by the appropriation of the body and reproductive processes of women by healthcare professionals, through inhumane treatment, abuse of medicalization and pathologizing of natural processes, causing the loss of autonomy and the ability to decide freely about their bodies, reproduction and sexuality, negatively affecting the quality of women's lives. (Parto do Principio, 2012)

A case of obstetric violence in Brazil

Adelir Carmen Lemos, a 29-year-old woman from the city of Torres in Rio Grande do Sul, wanted to have a normal birth for her third pregnancy, which had not been possible when she was pregnant with her first two children. Despite living in a country with the highest caesarean rates in the world (88% for those giving birth with private insurance and 52% for those without), she was looking forward to giving birth vaginally after previously having caesareans she felt were unnecessary. This time she had the support of a doula, her husband and the social movements that promote the rights of pregnant women and propagate evidence-based information. She found that, in other countries, a woman with one or more caesarean sections could plan to have a normal birth and that there are protocols for care in such cases. She also found out that for most Brazilian healthcare professionals such protocols are unknown and many believe that previous caesarean sections are absolute indications for a caesarean section in future births.

On 31st March 2014, Adelir went to the hospital where it was confirmed that her baby was fine. She was asked to sign a liability waiver stating that she preferred to avoid a caesarean section and allowing her to wait for labour at home. She knew that if she arrived at the hospital before labour was well established she would be forced to have a caesarean section. The doctor who attended her at the hospital disagreed with her decision and, arguing on behalf of the 'defence of the unborn child's life', sought legal prosecution, which triggered a court mandate. Court officials and armed policemen were sent to Adelir's home, and forced her to go back to the hospital. A caesarean section was performed against her wishes. The doctors believed that a vaginal birth would put Adelir and her baby at risk despite the evidence which shows that a caesarean would have been statistically more risky.

Adelir's case had international repercussions. It demonstrated an unacceptable disrespect to a woman's rights to autonomy, privacy, legality, and non-violence in contravention of international treaties. It also revealed serious violations of the Code of Medical Ethics such as a lack of consent without any imminent risk of death.

Humanization of care as public policy

Humanization of care is a buzzword in Brazil, and is the motto of the natural childbirth movement, which was born in the early 1990s. To humanize care is to provide effective care for all women, paying attention to psychological and physiological needs, and not resorting to medical technology. Humanized birth means putting the woman at the centre and in control so that she, and not the doctors, nurses, midwives or anyone else, makes the decisions about what will happen to her.

The movement for childbirth humanization is growing and getting stronger every day, yet local medical associations are fighting against it. Obstetricians are criticized and sometimes have been punished for heading up midwifery-led birth centres or for supporting the idea of home birth, each time provoking midwives, doulas and birthing women to fight back in the street, thus making the movement even more visible. The Brazilian Ministry of Health joined the cause and published a series of ministerial ordinances to promote safer motherhood programmes, humanize pregnancy, labour and birth care and implement birth centres.

All Brazilian states have now joined the Stork Network strategy, an initiative launched in March 2011 by the Ministry of Health as part of the Brazilian public healthcare system (Ministry Of Health Brazil, 2011). The Stork Network aims to ensure that all Brazilians receive appropriate, safe and humane care from confirmation of pregnancy, through antenatal and childbirth care, until the first two years of a baby's life. The Ministry of Health believes that women should have the right to reproductive planning and humanized assistance during pregnancy, childbirth, postpartum and abortion, and that children have the right to a safe birth, and healthy growth and development. The Ministry of Health has invested £3 billion in the scheme until 2014.

The role of social movements

The social movements of birth activists and feminists in Brazil proclaim: 'No more obstetric violence to sell caesarean sections'. Despite the prevailing belief in women's preference for caesarean sections, what women really want is to be free from abuse, abandonment, and neglect, preferably avoiding threats on their physical and sexual integrity. As long as the so-called 'normal birth' is attended aggressively and women are deprived of their rights, caesarean sections will appear less distressing, less painful and a safer alternative. It is an unfair choice between bad and worse, which is why so many women in the private sector appear to prefer caesarean sections.

The high caesarean birth rate recently sparked debates and protests in Brazil, which involved activists from organisations such as the NGO Parto do Princípio, who are opposed to the mode of childbirth being dictated by health insurance plans. Nevertheless, the reality of giving birth in Brazil's public – and especially private – hospitals does not correspond to this ideal. Obstetric violence is one of the greatest acts of disrespect for the rights of Brazilian women, and reflects the dehumanizing aspects of the healthcare system in Brazil.

Interventions that most healthcare professionals regard as 'normal', routine, everyday care (ie, episiotomy and oxytocin use without consent, birth lying on the back with the legs open, caesarean sections given for fictitious reasons) are now viewed by healthcare users as forms of obstetric violence. The gruesome reality of these procedures was exposed to much astonishment in the documentary *Obstetric violence – the voice of Brazilian women* (Zorzam *et al*, 2014).

Normal birth and humanized care, provided by birth professionals who are experienced and confident in providing care in physiological births, has become a consumerist ideal, a privilege only available for rich and educated women. However, in some parts of the country, women from the top of the social hierarchy prefer to use the public healthcare system to give birth precisely because this model of care is closer to the quality of care they desire.

It will require courage and boldness on the part of healthcare managers to change the aggressive and obsolete model that prevails. There needs to be a focus on the implementation of birth centres and the hiring of midwives and nurse-midwives so that healthy pregnant women can be cared for in the community. There should be increased interdisciplinary collaboration between maternity care teams. They should be integrated into the system with automatic access to the higher levels of complexity required if a transfer is needed. We need and deserve quality in the public healthcare SUS to differentiate it from the private sector, which still adheres to the undisguised model of unnecessary caesarean section for all.

Childbirth without violence, with respectful care and informed choice based on evidence is what should be offered to women.

Ana Paula and Clarissa's birth story

It was the longest 41 weeks of my life, particularly in the last weeks when I thought that time had stopped, and I would be eternally pregnant. It was a mix of anxiety and fear that I would have to suffer again. This feeling was devastating, since I'd already had the experience of pregnancy and birth, but did not bring my baby home. I was not afraid to suffer violence in childbirth care. I was afraid of another child dying before we got to meet her. I feared that the big date with her might also be the moment of farewell. I knew it was not healthy to feel like this and I really wanted to move on.

However, angels now surround us and as a couple we are brave enough to confront anyone in order to obtain respect. Information is everything. From the moment we heard the confirmation of pregnancy we decided to have a home birth. I did not want to have contact with the hospital environment at that moment of my life since it was fundamental to eliminate any trace of fear and the memory of my last delivery. I will only heal this trauma when I have my daughter in my arms.

We carried our pregnancy with love, good health and care, to ensure that the transition from inside to outside was also positive. Dr Lucas and the home birth midwives from Belo Horizonte led my antenatal care. My husband and I went happily to shower, singing and enjoying perhaps the last shower with Clarissa in my belly. We listened to music on our way to the hospital and we were greeted by Dr Lucas's calm smile. He introduced us to the midwife on call that night and told us that since the labour wards were unusually calm we would be admitted to the birth centre for induction of labour because he thought the home-like environment would be very helpful. Starting at eight o'clock that Sunday night until 2:50am the next day (the time of Clarissa's birth), I remember it was the greatest moment of my life. I believe that from the moment I set foot in the birth centre the world of 'partolândia' was presented to me.

At approximately 1am I was awakened by the frequent contractions of active labour. My midwife and a doula were beside me throughout labour and birth. The contractions came one after the other almost without intermission and seemed like a flood or a hurricane.

The contractions really are like waves and we must learn how to surf them. At times I would raise my arms as though I were standing up on a surfboard. Other times I took a hit from the waves, one of those that knock you down. And then, after a few minutes in the shower, I felt a strong push as if my whole body was bearing down. At that moment I regretted that I'd written in my birth plan that I didn't want anyone to touch me. I wanted to be hugged, but I had pushed everyone away like a cat that shudders whenever anyone touches it.

I looked at the door and someone invited me into the birth pool! Yay! The baby was coming! In there it was good because I had space around me. They rubbed grape seed oil on my back and threw water over me. I kept my eyes closed, and didn't know who was doing the massage. I just knew it felt good. But I could distinguish the touch of my husband André, who was rubbing my back.

Then came the moment of pushing the baby out, which I call when thunder and lightning meet. I felt as if lightning was coming down from the sky on top of my head, going through my entire body and ending in the vaginal canal. It was such a strong energy that I cannot describe it. I did not need to push Clarissa into the world because my body was working alone. I just needed to give in to myself, to surrender. And how it hurt!

Clarissa was born! Oh, what a relief! What pleasure! How wonderful! How magnificent! This feeling is awesome! It is immediate! The world stopped and I was in a state of grace, ecstatic with love. I had just given birth to my daughter. I was in love with Clarissa.

Where do we go from here?

The Ministry of Health (MoH) in Brazil sees the alarming high rates of caesarean sections as a major public health problem. However, the MoH acknowledges that the trivialization of caesarean sections to the point of being performed without need, the excessive use of interventions in labour and birth, and disrespect and abuse towards women's rights are trademarks of an intrinsic patriarchal society. By bringing all women into a hospital, childbirth has become a medical and surgical procedure. The MoH's challenge is to end the 'business' of birth by employing multidisciplinary care teams, where pregnancies considered low risk at the start of labour may be cared for by midwives in alongside and freestanding midwifery led-units so that an obstetrician is not solely responsible for labour and birth care. The implementation of maternity care environments that reduce the chances of medical interventions, respect women's autonomy and privacy, and increases maternal satisfaction should be respected in such a memorable event. There are those who believe that the most important factor in maternity care is for the baby to be born healthy, no matter what. For others, however, the way we give birth has a profound impact on the human race.

KEY MESSAGES

- Significant progress has been made in maternal and neonatal healthcare in Brazil. Despite these improvements, access to quality maternity services is not guaranteed.
- The abuse of unnecessary interventions, such as acceleration of labour with synthetic oxytocin and caesarean sections, has been associated with higher morbidity and mortality to both mother and baby.
- Overlapping with the humanization of childbirth movement, and with increasing momentum for respectful maternity care globally, is the social and political movement to eliminate obstetric violence in Brazil.

ACTION POINTS

- Obstetrics is the art of caring for women in difficult and complicated births, not disrupting physiological labour, and surgically delivering the baby once birthing via the natural canal is rendered impossible.
- Strengthen midwifery so that midwives have the autonomy to be primary care providers in partnership with women and their families.
- Maternity care workers should adopt an approach based on evidence, centred on the individual, based on principles of ethics and respect for human rights, and promote practices that recognize women's preferences and women's and newborns' needs.
- Make improvements in the healthcare system, such as strengthening facility infrastructure and commodities, providing adequate staffing and resources, and avoiding human resource shortages that may contribute to provider burn-out, demoralization and thus disrespectful or abusive care.
- Increase awareness among pregnant women and families of their rights, healthy practices during pregnancy, labour and birth, implementing community activities, including campaigns about women's rights in childbirth.

21 Making it happen in Catalonia, Spain

Ramón Escuriet *Translation* Roberto Ortíz

The Spanish National Health System includes childbirth, delivery and post-partum care in its health services portfolio. Childbirth is one of the most common reasons for admission to Catalonian hospitals. Over the last decades Catalonian hospitals have been developing new and advanced techniques aiming to improve the quality of care of women and to deal with newly identified complications during delivery. Nowadays, and perhaps due to these improvements, we have achieved very good results and high-quality standards in maternal and perinatal health, but this has come at a cost, in terms of increasing rates of intervention in labour and birth in some settings. This chapter examines the nature and impact of a new policy-led approach to improve the quality of care for childbearing women in Catalonia.

A new strategy for maternity care in Catalonia

Over the last few years, childbirth care within the public health system has become the centre of attention of the Catalonian health administration. As a consequence, the National Health Ministry has elaborated a new Strategy to promote natural childbirth in the public hospitals. In contrast to the largely medically led maternity service that currently exits, this new Strategy has proposed that the midwife should be the lead professional for women anticipating and experiencing normal childbirth.

Two main factors have influenced this strategic change. On the one hand, it is driven by the active participation of women who want to be in charge of their own decisions regarding the type of care they prefer during childbirth and delivery. On the other, public administration bodies have become concerned about the adverse outcomes of routine interventions carried out without any appropriate justification in childbirth care, and the financial, personal and societal costs of these interventions.

How to motivate change through implementation of public health policies

Any change in the health system is a major challenge for public health administrations. To ensure that this is undertaken efficiently and effectively, the Catalan Department of Health decided to start a new project for the implementation of good practices in childbirth. The three main aims were to improve the existing hospital infrastructure, to optimize clinical practice, and to improve information for maternity service users so that they could increase their capacity to make informed decisions about their care in childbirth, delivery and postpartum, based on their individual values, beliefs and circumstances. All these actions were developed simultaneously, and have been implemented gradually since 2008. Specifically, the Department of Health allocated an improvement budget to designated hospitals, and identified a manager at each location, who would be responsible for ensuring that the budget was spent appropriately to meet the needs of their particular hospital in terms of delivering the Strategy.

All hospitals participating in this project were recognized and their names published in the Catalan Health Service annual list.

Achievements so far

At the time of writing, there are 32 hospitals recognized in the Service List (out of 43 public hospitals in Catalonia). All are working together to implement good practice in normal birth care. Fourteen have incorporated birthing pools onto their labour wards. Some have created home-like rooms/areas where women experiencing spontaneous labour and birth can stay. As well as birthing pools, these areas include inexpensive additions, such as birthing balls, and soft lighting, to promote a relaxed atmosphere during labour and birth. Anecdotally, this has created a welcoming environment for maternity care staff as well as for maternity service users. The audit evidence that is emerging suggests that these changes have catalyzed the implementation of best practice recommendations in childbirth, as well as contributing to a reduction in routine intrapartum interventions.

Alongside these changes in hospital infrastructure, new clinical guidance for normal childbirth has been produced, and several recommendations for natural childbirth care have been disseminated among all health professionals, with the intention of helping them to abandon routine and unjustified practices, and to implement practices based on scientific evidence. Midwifery and obstetric associations have been funded by the Catalonian Department of Health to offer official study days free of charge for everybody who wants to attend them. These study days are orientated to natural childbirth care, leadership and research, to promote and achieve good clinical practice, and respectful maternity care provision.

Well known and recognized local health professionals have collaborated to elaborate this new clinical guidance to encourage their adoption and implementation into clinical practice. After publishing the recommendations, a new research project was initiated. It started with the collaboration of a number of health professionals who had different points of view of natural birth, with the main objective of working towards a new clinical practice consent form. This, along with all the other documents arising from the project, has been uploaded to the Department of Health website.

In 2009, a series of open days were held for maternity care professionals on the topic of natural childbirth care. The content included relevant recommendations made by the Health Department as well as innovative new practices that had been developed both in Catalonia and internationally. Service users also came to tell their stories. As one said: 'I wish for health professionals to hear about my own doubts and anxieties, to be informed, and to be able to choose.'

These open days were attended by 350 health professionals (midwives and obstetricians).

Informed choice by women is the key to changing outdated attitudes to healthcare. It was therefore considered very important to develop a birthing and delivery plan to aid communication between service users and health professionals. This is also available on the official Department of Health website, so that any woman can download and complete it, and present it to any Catalonian public hospital when they are admitted in labour. Many hospitals have developed and adapted their own documents with the purpose of informing women about what can be offered on their labour ward. This development work has often included both hospital and community health providers, creating an exceptional opportunity to co-ordinate maternity care across these settings.

What is changing?

This section tells a personal story of how the project started, and then presents personal reflections on what it has achieved.

(November 2007) The baby had just started to breastfeed, her mother was tired but happy to hold her baby in her arms, and then I left the room quietly. It had been an intense night on duty. A few hours later, while I was at home, the sound of the phone woke me up. An important project to improve maternity care in the Spanish National Health System was going to be launched, and I was going to work on it!

My experience as a midwife for 15 years would help me in this challenge, but I also had to learn about management and health economics. The priority for the public health administration is implementing best practices and to improve maternity care within the national health system, and my responsibility to date is to carry it out in Catalonia. After several years working on the project, this chapter gives me the opportunity to share some of my best lived experiences so that this may help others who are working to improve health care of women and their families.

(August 2014) Many actions have been done up to date and many health professionals are participating in this project. New initiatives are arising, and many concerns and perceptions have emerged. Meeting with health professionals and visiting the hospitals is helpful as a way of identifying what has been done so far and what remains to be done. But, can we really say that things are changing, or is it only my personal perception? What do other colleagues think about it?

'I can still remember when I had to hide from other colleagues to help mothers to put babies skin-to-skin after birth… now everything has changed, skin-to-skin is normal for everybody, mothers do ask to be with their babies and all midwives do promote it.'… 'I'm now retired, but during my last working days I felt that I could work peacefully…' Lourdes Martínez, Senior Midwife.

'I've seen many changes in labour wards during these last years. Some time ago it was impossible not to separate the newborn from the mother, it was impossible to take and respect the necessary time for each stage of labour, also impossible to allow women to adopt different positions during labour or during childbirth. All these things are now part of the past! We can now establish a special relationship with women during childbirth, sometimes we are complicit with them, so we can laugh, or weep emotionally together… I think these incoming changes are helping us to improve our work and also to become better midwives.' Vanesa Bueno, Hospital Midwife

What about infrastructure? Is it worthwhile investing in buying new material or reshaping labour wards to make spaces more comfortable?

'You know that this is a little hospital and women didn't feel like coming here was the best option either for them, or for their babies. Since we have this new room with the bath…. we can work better, we can offer different options to women, they can use water during labour and we can really feel that we are working as midwives. Now women living in this area know that we are doing things differently and they want to come here.' Montse Bach, Hospital Midwife

Many midwives and some obstetricians have been participating in training activities. How do professionals perceive this and how is this impacting on day to day practice?

'For a long time we have been working to provide warm care to all women during childbirth, and we have been receiving midwives from other units who wanted to learn how we are working here. It was fantastic and a great recognition to be invited within this Project to show our work in these study days: some of those midwives who attended the study days are now coming back to us telling their positive experiences.' Alicia Ferrer, Midwife Supervisor

Other main concerns come from the continuing clinical practice variability and the information provided to women to promote autonomous decision making. Are we all doing and explaining the same things?

'It has been very rewarding to leave the "Tower of Babel" that had become antenatal and childbirth care. Now the midwives speak the same language with which we advise the pregnant woman to prepare her own birth plan and we can also accompany her to make it a reality... always respecting their decisions.' Xavi Espada, Hospital and Community Midwife

'We have all the necessary technology and we can immediately act if it is necessary, but only if it is necessary! We really think (all the health professional team) that our main job is to support the normal development of labour and birth as a physiological process, without unnecessary interventions. Since we work this way we have also found that intervention levels in our obstetric unit have decreased...' Joan Meléndez, Obstetrician and President of the Advisory Commission for Maternal Health of the Department of Health

A great deal of support was found from midwives' representatives in all activities promoted by the Department of Health and some of them have been closely working on the project, motivating and supporting midwives and midwifery students to implement best practices and to promote a woman-focused model of care.

'We are aware that society perceptions about our profession and ethics has changed since this Project was launched. Such changes have also helped to encourage women's rights and respect. As midwives, we have regained our professional autonomy within the health teams, and we can demonstrate our efficiency as health professionals. From a global perspective we can also say that the Project is helping us to improve our clinical practice and regain the essence of our profession, and in consequence we are positively contributing to improve the current maternity model of care and women's health... We can now assume that we are a reference professional for women along the sexual and reproductive health of women.' Isabel Salgado, Chair of Midwives in the College of Nurses

'It is exciting to learn to become a midwife, one of the most ancient professions of humankind that midwives have taught to me as an art. They taught me to be beside the woman, to take care of her and to be with her during the exciting journey of pregnancy. My way to become a midwife has been full of emotions from my very first day. All births that I've seen and attended have made me feel alive. I could feel that it was the closest and most sensitive contact with life and even with death! Now as a young and recently graduated midwife, I can put into practice all the teachings received from my mentors (now colleagues). I can only be grateful for all their support helping me in my "birth" as a midwife...'
Georgina Picas, Recently Graduated Midwife

Conclusion

The policy-led project described in this chapter has turned childbirth in general, and natural birth in particular, into a priority for Catalonian health policies and hospitals, and has made the citizens of Catalonia aware of the importance of childbirth to society. Infrastructure improvements have created spaces that are much more comfortable for labouring women and provided the possibility for them to use birthing pools during birth, as well as offering them positive information, and building up their confidence in their capacity to labour and give birth.

All of this has motivated health professionals to initiate more local projects to implement good practice in hospitals, and in some of these initiatives hospital staff have started to work together with community health services.

Within the framework of the new Strategy, new conditions have been created regarding the structure of maternity care, professional practice, and the way in which women participate in their own labour and birth process. The changes observed so far indicate a deep change, including rethinking of a more comprehensive model of maternity care in which childbirth is considered as a physiological process requiring respectful care without unnecessary interventions.

This model of maternity care re-orientation is leading to a re-organization of health professional teams, and is also having a positive effect on the way midwives and obstetricians interact professionally. Women are now participating more actively during the whole process, in the context of more comfortable rooms for childbirth where they can have freedom of movement, accompaniment by a relative, and continuous professional support.

It is hoped that the successes so far may increase the potential for further achievements, so that the changes observed to date can continue to evolve into the future.

KEY MESSAGES

- The Catalonian government realized that something had to be done to decrease rising rates of routine intervention in labour.
- A new maternity care strategy was developed, including improvements to labour and birth infrastructure, such as the addition of birthing pools; staff education in how to maximize normal childbirth; increased collaboration between hospital and community care provision; and community engagement through specific initiatives like online downloadable birth plans.
- Evaluation of the new strategy indicated that some interventions were reduced, with no adverse effects on wellbeing, and increased reports of maternal and staff wellbeing.

ACTION POINTS

- Policy makers who want to make a difference in maternity care need to analyze the existing situation, explore variability in clinical practice, and prioritize actions to improve maternity care provision, especially normal birth care.
- Service providers need to develop the necessary conditions to facilitate best practice implementation. This could include initial investment to promote structural changes, increase awareness by maternity health professionals, and encourage women's participation and decision making in their own maternity care process.
- Continuous support, co-ordination, evaluation and dissemination from the lead policy maker are essential for the implementation and promotion of new initiatives. This needs to include service providers, health professionals, women using the service, and local communities.
- Maternity professionals should always keep in mind that they are a 'lucky guest' in one of the most special moments in the life of a woman who is giving birth. This is an exceptional opportunity to create the optimal conditions for a warm welcome to the life of a newborn and to positively contribute to this experience. Compassionate care can always be provided, and technical paraphernalia should be used rationally, and only when it is clearly necessary.
- Listen respectfully. Women's expectations should always be considered during all labour and birth processes.

22 Italy, where is your beauty?

Laura Iannuzzi and Sandra Morano

Italy represents an 'exceptional' country for many very good reasons, but one unwelcome area in which Italy leads is, sadly, our caesarean section (CS) rate. Estimated at around 38% of all births, it represents the highest rate in Europe and one of the highest in the world (Ministero della Salute, 2011). In achieving such a record of CS, a significant role has been played by a culture that has progressively led women to believe that they have lost their birthing capacity, making them, their families, attending professionals and society as a whole abnormally anxious and fearful about childbirth. Though other maternity systems worldwide have been influenced by this medically dominated culture of fear and a birth technology market (Reiger and Dempsey, 2006), the fruits of obstetric surgery have flourished particularly quickly and abundantly in Italy.

Despite this challenging scenario, both small and larger counter-revolutions have happened in our country. These transformations have been as much about personal change as about our professional development. We wanted to share something of the stories behind these changes, where the presence of – or desire for – kindness, compassion, respect and courage has made the difference.

Personal narratives, challenges, and revolutions: discovering ourselves, so near, so far

Sandra

My narrative begins with the birth of my sister at home, at a time when children were not allowed to participate. But my influences can be traced back to my grandmother's 14 births: 12 girls, and two boys who died at birth. It was the story of my country, and of the women in between the two World Wars, when maternity still had an important meaning in communities and giving birth was a part of life.

At the end of my journey at medical school (the late 1970s), labouring women, and midwives along with them, had already been banished from homes in Italy for a decade. The long history of help between women within homes was annihilated with the introduction of hospital births. It was the sign of the technology of modern times, the promise of civilization, and a tangible example of the fight against materno-fetal mortality. Science did the rest. Healthy childbearing women's bodies were made to conform to the healthcare discipline. Midwives were transformed into jailers; specialized obstetricians replaced the old practitioners and gained high visibility. The languages of maternal solidarity and the traditional symbols of procreation were swept away and relegated to heirlooms of illiteracy. Those of us training to be obste-

tricians at the time encountered industrialized childbearing women coming to the hospital, placed alone on a bed in a labour room, and being forced to leave their husbands and family out of the delivery suite.

At that time many of us rebelled: we were labelled bad students. We had to decide how to learn about birth, what to learn and, above all, whose side to be on. We were of course on the side of the women, and so we intuitively rejected what we were required to do. We could not rebuke women who were shouting because they were being forced to go through labour tied to a CTG (cardiotocography), pushing supine, having episiotomy by default and so on. Instead, we chose to leave, to look for like-thinking practitioners, and to fight. We started to travel, from south to north, around Italy first, and then Europe. We rejected the teachings, the tranquillity of tyranny, and the cosiness of a 'simple' execution of orders. Disobeying. We looked for other models, in anthropology, psychoanalysis, gynaecology and paediatrics. We had encounters at conferences. We had personal fights in labour wards just to save one woman from an inappropriate episiotomy. We had arguments with colleagues, with important and authoritative professors and sometimes with depersonalized midwives, and almost reached the very edge of sadism. We were many, though few compared to the bulk. Changing, changing, changing. Times, practices, places. Those places that marked the otherness of women from their bodies, from their ancestral intimate certainties.

Laura

I was just born in the 1970s, but I inherited and experienced much of the 1970s culture. Indeed, during my training as a midwife in the 1990s in Florence, the majority of those practices, now openly questioned, were still routinely performed and taught.

I used to blame the doctors exclusively for the over-medicalization of birth, but soon discovered that the culture I was questioning was the result of more complex dynamics with several actors, me included. In this regard, I would never forget the time when a woman lying semi-recumbent in bed in her second stage kindly asked: 'Laura, but why can't I push on my side?' Right, why? I had no reasons except for 'hospital rules'. By simply posing a question she helped me to unveil what was there but I couldn't see: I was strongly immersed in the system I didn't like. While provoking my reflexivity she gave to me what I was supposed to offer her: compassion, empowerment, care. As you might guess, she ended up giving birth to her baby the way she wanted. I realized then that to change an environment, a system, a culture, I needed to change first.

My personal revolution started silently. It was a slow process of mutation with some clamorous 'points of no return'. One of those has a specific name: Tricia Anderson. I met Tricia in 2003 during a course on physiological birth in Florence. At that time, many Italian midwives were advocating for normal births, but encountering Tricia actually challenged and fascinated me as never before. She was

such an extraordinary witness to the beauty of childbirth and midwifery in practice,
education and research. And beauty is a catalyst for change. She provided convinc-
ing rationales for each statement; her knowledge was remarkable and amazingly
communicated. She offered lots of 'tricks' to use to modify the system. That was
key as motivation is fundamental but you also need to see the feasibility of a goal
in order to avoid frustration. She questioned and blamed practices rather than the
professionals who carried them out. Ultimately, she made me feel not only 'part of
the problem' but 'part of the solution', whereas hospital midwives seemed bad mid-
wives by definition. I started seeking possibilities for change everywhere, supporting
colleagues in the daily battles and building critical collaborations.

Snapshots from Italian birth centres

Our different journeys led us to work in two of the few birth centres in Italy. There are so few because a highly medicalized culture like the Italian
one is keen to maintain the status quo, and rarely promotes woman-centred and midwifery-led models of care. Yet, despite the difficulties, these
birth centres have started to open up, offering wonders for families and
maternity care providers, while provoking a scandalized reaction from
the Italian maternity system.

Centro Nascita Alternativo (CNA), the 'alternative' birth centre attached to the San Martino University Hospital in Genoa, was the first
alongside birth centre in Italy. It was created by Sandra and a strong group
of midwives in 2000, and even the name was considered a scandal. The
staff received a kind of 'reverse training', which was designed to reorien-
tate them to the physiology of labour and birth. The development of this
training programme was aided by Susanne Houd. The 'Margherita' birth
centre (Centro Nascita Margherita) has operated since 2007 alongside
the Careggi University Hospital in Florence. Initially planned by a doctor, it opened, after fervent debates, as the first midwife-led unit in Italy
headed by a midwife, Rita Breschi. Passion, resilience, trust, respect and
good results have been fundamental ingredients of its midwifery team.

These places appeared scandalous because they offered colourful
home-like environments within university hospitals, cradles of 'high-tech'
knowledge, bringing back midwives as the lead carers for women in the
public health system. They became territories of 'compromises' between
home and hospitals, and so were unacceptable for many observers. They
witnessed conflicts between different professional groups (McCourt *et
al*, 2014), but they also catalyzed strong alliances between colleagues and
women, and introduced different worldviews. They are places where the
courage of the few has become the courage of the many. They increasing-

ly invaded their neighbourhoods, becoming crucial in influencing and supporting other units in Italy, but gaining also an international reputation. They encourage reflexivity and compassion at the same level as good clinical practice, allowing for the use of both evidence-based protocols, and for the flexibility in using them (or not) to meet women's needs.

Including compassion as an element of care opens up the possibility of experiencing the wonder of birth. This is apparent every time the eligibility of women to attend the birth centre is discussed by the staff team.

Sandra

I want to use this story as an example of compassion in action.

Two years ago a woman with a lymphoma in remission asked to give birth in the CNA birth centre, raising long discussions among midwives on whether she could meet the 'low-risk' criteria. I thought 'In what way could childbirth affect her illness?' I met the woman when she was waiting for her labour, and she was fine. In my opinion she was manifestly a 'low-risk' mother. In the event, the midwife said this woman gave birth wonderfully and was happy and confident in taking care of her baby. When I visited her after the birth, she told me: 'I've experienced what illness, risk, desperation and pain is. What had I to be afraid of? I did feel this was the only place where I could experience the beauty of normal birth.'

Conclusion: beauty is a catalyst for change

Birth centres are often described as flagships of the Italian maternity system, yet their establishment and existence is constantly threatened, regardless of their excellent outcomes, women's satisfaction, and the evidence base. By reading mothers' messages or looking at parents who revisit these places just to make sure they will be there, available, for their next baby, we can understand why we have to keep defending and promoting such places in Italy. Their science, respect, creativity must be protected and nourished. The truth is, those who oppose these models have not yet fully understood the importance of their existence, and of the philosophy of care that animates them, of their testimony to the beauty of birth. We still have to fight for this to be grasped. The truth is, *we need beauty*, and even more concerning childbirth. We must not be tired of looking for systems of maternity care that are beautiful in their capacity to maximize positive attitudes and behaviours, and wellbeing and optimum labour and birth for women, their families, and the staff who attend them. Once such beauty is found, we must not be tired of safeguarding it.

KEY MESSAGES

- Despite the challenging scenario of the Italian maternity system, and particularly the high caesarean section rate, counter-revolutions have happened. Nothing is impossible.
- The need for change is as much about professional values, attitudes, beliefs and behaviours as about the settings in which people work.
- Beauty is a catalyst for change.

ACTION POINTS

- Don't always look for 'external' enemies. Start the revolution from yourself.
- Listen to women: even a woman's simple question can reawaken an unreflective professional.
- Every little change matters: think big, but start with small steps.
- Provide a rationale for every choice, and motivate but also lead others to see the feasibility of a goal.
- Seek alliances, and find inspirational fellow travellers.
- Support those who share your daily battles.

23 A good birth in the Netherlands

Raymond De Vries, Marijke Hendrix, Tamar van Haaren
and the members of the Midwifery Science Workgroup

The Dutch are widely known for their well-integrated maternity care system where autonomous midwives care for the majority of women and where women can freely choose between birth at home, in a polyclinic, or in hospital. Such choices tend to optimize individualized respectful maternity care. This chapter examines whether the Dutch way of birth is a vestige of the past or the vanguard of the future (De Vries et al, 2009).

Maternity care in the Netherlands

The 19th-century German poet Heinrich Heine is reported to have said *'When the world comes to an end, I shall go to Holland, for everything there happens fifty years later.'* This statement is the source of some bemusement among the Dutch, and has been used both to celebrate and to decry maternity care in the Netherlands. Some protagonists proudly note that, if being fifty years behind means having a sensible approach to birth care that avoids the unnecessary medicalization of birth, empowers women, reduces the rate of surgical births, and decreases infant and maternal morbidity, then being behind actually means being ahead of the rest of the world. Others use Heine's statement to criticize Dutch maternity care as 'old-fashioned' – 'something from the middle ages' – declaring that it is time for the Netherlands to catch up with its neighbours by framing maternity care provision with an obstetric philosophy, and by bringing all births into the hospital. Regardless of one's opinion about maternity care in the Netherlands, it is a system based on the principle that pregnancy and childbirth are fundamentally physiological processes. Given that principle, midwives who are independent of medical supervision provide care to healthy women with uncomplicated pregnancies. They refer women to obstetric-led care only when there is an increased risk of complications as defined by the 'List of Obstetric Indications' (LOI), a national guideline developed co-operatively by all the professions involved in maternity care. Women with a healthy pregnancy are free to follow their preferences and give birth at home or in a hospital-based polyclinic setting under the supervision of their midwife. In midwifery-led care, women will not receive medical interventions such as pharmacological pain relief, labour augmentation, or continuous fetal monitoring, unless they need referral to obstetric-led care.

The physiological orientation towards birth that is inherent in Dutch maternity care is underscored by the national policy mandating that healthy women who choose to give birth in the polyclinic must make a co-payment of approximately €300 for the additional costs of the hospital stay. Built into this regulation is the notion that healthy women, as defined by the LOI, can (and should) have their babies at home.

The uniqueness of the Dutch maternity care system has made it a model for those who seek to slow or reverse the march towards the routine use of interventions in birth that is found in most countries around the world (van Teijlingen *et al*, 2004). Although the Dutch maternity care system is experiencing change that is pushing in the direction of more routine intervention, including increased pressure to bring midwives under medical supervision (De Vries *et al*, 2013), the Netherlands remains an important destination for birth activists who wish to maximize respectful and dignified maternity care by learning how to reorganize and demedicalize birth in their home countries.

Stories of maternity care in the Netherlands

Too often descriptions of the Dutch way of birth are limited to statistical portrayals of caregivers and outcomes. While these are clearly necessary, they exclude the voices of maternity care givers, and of the women and families they serve, and they fail to convey what occurs in the homes, polyclinics, and hospitals of the Netherlands. Listening to these voices provides an understanding of why the Dutch system inspires those who seek to reduce the medical aspects of the human event of birth. Here are two accounts of birth in the Netherlands, the first told by a mother about her second birth:

My second pregnancy was not as exciting as my first, I was often tired and had many colds. [My labour began when] I felt a weak contraction, and then a while later, another small one. I decided to go to bed nice and early. If I could get to sleep, maybe the contractions would stop. That did not work. I was definitely having contractions, so I went with my big bare belly and stood in front of the gas heater. That felt great! The contractions became stronger and more regular and we called the midwife.

First came the assistant and then the midwife. My friend Jetske came with a big bouquet of fragrant lilies. My neighbour, Otto, happened to come by and asked if he could stay. Sure, why not? Between contractions I was able to relax, and when another came I was able to handle it easily. I felt like an old hand at this. Gradually the contractions became more frequent and intense and I suddenly recalled how vicious some contractions can be.

I began to feel irritated and impatient. I had had enough of this, I wanted no more. Soon came the urge to push but I had to keep these strong contractions at a distance, I had to puff them away. But they were so powerful I had to go along with them, and when I did I found that I enjoyed them. The midwife broke the membranes. And then, an enormous relief, my second child arrived, a beautiful little girl with dark hair, Rosa.

She lay next to me safe and warm, softly groaning as if gradually recovering from her journey. When everyone had gone and Frans, my husband, was sleeping on the sofa and Swaan, my little daughter, was in her bed, and Rosa in my arms, the room changed into an island of rest, the center of the universe (Spanier et al, 1994, pp366–367).

From the point of view of a childbearing woman, this story illustrates both the normality and the extraordinary nature of birth when it is conducted in an environment that maximizes respectful relationships and compassionate care.

The second story comes from the point of view of the midwife. Here, Beatrijs Smulders, a practising midwife in the Netherlands, highlights the advantages of the Dutch way of birth for women, from her perspective of having observed many births over many years:

A good birth strengthens the self-image of the birthing woman at a deep, non-rational level. A system in which women do the delivery themselves emancipates women. Often women say after the delivery: 'After this I can do anything!' or 'Because I was forced to rely on myself during the delivery, I learned all of a sudden to trust myself.'

This is well illustrated by the story of a professor, whose pregnancy at the age of 43 was unexpected and unwanted. She never had the desire to have children. She had, in fact, achieved everything that a woman could achieve in a 'man's world'. She was a university professor, had written bestsellers, and was on several important policy committees. And then this, totally unexpected! At her prenatal visits she was often confused, not knowing whether to be happy or grief-stricken. She worked harder than ever, and she wanted to return to work as soon as possible after the delivery. She was not looking forward to the birth. This cool-headed woman preferred to go to hospital with plenty of pain relief. She questioned why we midwives were so keen on the use of water – being under the shower or in the bath during contractions. To her that seemed totally ridiculous. Her mind was made up and I promised to respect her wishes.

But during the pregnancy she changed – she followed a parent-craft course, attended an antenatal education evening and during the last check-up she suggested that: 'the first few centimetres dilation I'll stay at home, and well, the pain relief can come at the end'.

Her delivery started slowly. She found it extremely difficult to put aside the troubling thoughts that filled her head and to give in to her contractions, to her body. When she finally let go, the delivery went unbelievably fast. She insisted on staying at home, and even hopped into the 'damned' bath. She dilated fully and within an hour she had a beautiful son in her arms.

Six weeks later she came for her postpartum check-up. She was a very different person, in one arm her son breastfeeding, in the other a big bunch of roses. When I asked her to reflect on her birth she glowed and said: 'For years I have fought to make it in a man's world. Even though I succeeded something essential was missing. Now that I have had a baby, I know what that is. At a very deep level I was always unsure about myself, now something fundamental has changed. Rationally I can't put my finger on it, but bodily, intuitively, I have a new self-esteem that I had never experienced before, and as a result I am certain that that everything will become easier for me.'

This is the kind of reason that makes it so crucial that we in the Netherlands must hold onto a maternity care system that allows women, as much as possible, to make their own decisions and take control over pregnancy and birth, a system where women can choose their own midwife and take things into their own hands.

Conclusion

These stories of good births in the Netherlands demonstrate the value of reducing the technical aspects of pregnancy and birth that have removed the mother from the experience and diminished the opportunity for birth to enrich the lives of mothers, fathers, and families. That these stories originate in the Netherlands is a reminder that the way birth care is organized there is fundamental to the promotion of good births, births where the mother feels safe, cared for, and respected for who she is as a person. This kind of care is possible in the Netherlands because women recognize that birth is not a medical event and they have the opportunity to choose where and how their babies will be born; midwives have the autonomy they need to provide a 'midwife model of care' where medical interventions are used only when necessary; and obstetricians/gynaecologists recognize that their skills are not needed by women who have healthy pregnancies and births.

KEY MESSAGES

- A good birth strengthens the self-image of the birthing woman at a deep, non-rational level.
- Whilst statistical portrayals of childbirth maternity care workers and

the outcomes are useful, their voices, and those of the women and families they serve, are equally as important.

- Listening to care providers and childbearing women provides an understanding of why the Dutch system inspires those who seek to increase respectful, caring and compassionate aspects of the human event of childbirth, through optimizing women's capacity for physiological labour and birth.

ACTION POINTS

- Educators, policy makers and professionals should work on the cultural level to
  (a) alter cultural images that 'catastrophize' birth, and that teach women that birth is frightening and dangerous;
  (b) inform young women (preferably before they enter secondary school) about the physiology of birth and teach them that birth is a normal, healthy life event.
- Childbearing women, policy makers, maternity service designers, and practitioners should work on the structural level to
  (a) support midwives by working for legislation that gives them the autonomy to practise independently, as well as supporting respectful interprofessional relationships
  (b) let your local hospital know how important it is to have midwife-led care available to all women, in conjunction with effective and mutually respectful interdisciplinary referral mechanisms where these are necessary.

24 Open disclosure: a perspective from Ireland

Deirdre Munro

Maternity services in Ireland are experiencing an extremely troublesome period. Tragic incidents specific to Irish maternity care are consistently exposed in the media. Women, their partners and families frequently question the ability of our maternity services. Healthcare professionals work under stressful conditions leading to exhaustion and increasing anxiety, which facilitates a breeding ground of negativity and fear. Could this epidemic of fear be curtailed if confidence and positivity are given an opportunity to flourish? Where do we begin? Perhaps embracing 'open disclosure' provides a start to build the basic foundations of an open, safer, stronger maternity service. This chapter provides a brief overview of open disclosure, identifies international case studies, and shares key practical points of learning gained in these early days of openness in Ireland.

What is open disclosure?

Literature defines 'open disclosure' as the prompt, open, consistent, compassionate and honest communication with patients and families when a healthcare incident results in harm (MCPME, 2006; ACSQHC, 2008a; NPSA, 2009). This includes expressing regret for what has happened, keeping the patient informed, providing feedback on investigations and the steps taken to prevent a reoccurrence of the adverse event (MCPME, 2006).

Openness, honesty and transparency should be an 'always event' with each individual episode of care, within and between each department and in each and every organization.

The UK National Patient Safety Agency (NPSA, 2009a) refers to open disclosure as 'being open', describing a set of principles that healthcare staff should use when communicating with patients, their families and carers following an incident involving patient safety. Communication and introductions provide a golden key to unlock deeper compassionate care and need to start at the very beginning. Dr Kate Granger, a campaigning doctor, an advocate and a patient with terminal cancer, explains in her own words: 'During a hospital stay last summer I made the stark observation that many staff looking after me did not introduce themselves before delivering care. This felt very wrong so encouraged and supported by my husband we decided to start a campaign to encourage and remind healthcare staff about the importance of introductions in the delivery of care. I firmly believe it is not just about knowing someone's name, but it runs much deeper. It is about making a human connection, beginning a therapeutic relationship and building trust. In my mind it is the first rung on the ladder to providing compassionate care'. Kate is the founder of the #hellomynameis campaign (Granger, 2014).

When things go wrong in healthcare ideally openness, honesty, kindness and compassion should continue. However, immediately after an adverse event, the window of opportunity, which Dr Albert Wu refers to as the 'golden hour for disclosure', all too often vanishes due to defensiveness, damage limitation attempts and the fear of reputational damage. A preventable injury is also an injury to the patient's trust, and to the relationship. Each day that passes without effective communication adds harm to the patient and family (Wu, 2010). In addition to the human cost, financial implications for organizations are significant. Three case studies illustrate the benefits of open disclosure. The Mater Hospital in Brisbane, Australia, achieved a reduction in claims over a four-year period, saving $2 million AUD, following the introduction of open disclosure (Wu, 2009a). The Singapore Academic Hospital saved approximately $500,000 SGD per year, and zero cases preceded to litigation over a two-year period (Wu, 2009b). The University of Michigan Hospital experienced law suits being halved, saving an average of $2 million US dollars (Boothman *et al*, 2009).

Open disclosure in Ireland

The National Standards for Safer Better Healthcare (HIQA, 2012) state that 'service providers fully and openly inform and support service users as soon as possible after an adverse event affecting them has occurred, or becomes known and continue to provide information and support as needed'.

Between October 2010 and October 2012 the Health Service Executive National Advocacy Unit piloted an open disclosure programme at two hospitals, the Mater Misericordiae University Hospital Dublin and Cork University Maternity Hospital. Utilizing the learning from the pilot programme a national policy and national guidelines on open disclosure were developed in conjunction with the State Claims Agency. A patient information leaflet, staff support booklet and staff briefing guide were produced as supporting documents and launched on 12th November 2013. At the time of writing the policy was being evaluated.

A reality check

In reality staff express intense shock and fear following an adverse event. I have personally experienced those feelings of horror and denial, blaming myself and colleagues, experiencing perceived whispering and finger pointing, and being angry with myself at the loss of situational control. I have walked in those shoes of sheer isolation.

Following a recent midwifery evaluation of open disclosure one midwife expressed a 'lack of control' and remarked 'the majority of midwives are always open and honest with information on the frontline but if something big happens then clinical managers, directors or the legal team often control further communication and take over...' (All Ireland Midwifery Conference, 2014).

The literature identifies staff involved in an adverse event as the 'second victim' (Wu, 2000). This vulnerability is also evident as a senior midwife shared her story 'the media makes us out as monsters and we need someone to defend us to the public, we need support now more than ever... so who is there for the staff?' (All Ireland Midwifery Conference, 2014). Fear of litigation and loss of registration is also reported. This is the stark reality for practitioners on the ground. Deeper channels of communication need to occur between Irish legal practitioners and healthcare policymakers to review current Irish legislation.

Should an adverse event occur it is helpful to walk in the midwife's shoes. Everyone is in shock; the midwife is immediately the 'second victim' (Wu, 2000). As well as a personal journey of coping, a midwife is possibly exposed to the following expedition of enquiries:

Coroner's Court, Internal Enquiry, External Enquiry, Health Information Quality Authority Investigation, High Court, Preliminary Fitness to Practice, Full Fitness to Practice, European Court, as well as trial by colleagues and media. This is often compounded by a deafening silence from work colleagues and the void of support obviously needed to support staff.

What can I do?

A starting point in cases involving unintentional harm to patients is openness, kindness and mutual support. Having an open door, an open ear, and just being there without judgement can provide a shoulder to lean on and could possibly change a person's world. Listening, hearing and acting if necessary and always respecting your colleagues' confidentiality leads to a trusting relationship. Empathy can be promoted by imagining for one second how traumatic it is to walk in those shoes.

The support of professional organizations such as the Irish Nurses and Midwives Organization and the Royal College of Midwives often lacks appreciation, yet is clearly critical to a midwife. A recent evaluation of midwives' views of open disclosure identified a further 'need for peer support from another colleague having experienced an adverse event as well as specific input from our union' (All Ireland Midwifery Conference, 2014).

Conclusion

Midwives and doctors already recognize the need for systemic change in maternity services. Clear communication within maternity services is essential. The goodwill and best intentions of all staff need to be nurtured and valued. The acceptance of unintentional harm allows adverse events to be dealt with honestly, openly and compassionately. Should an incident occur to you or a member of your own family, how would you like to be treated? Disclosure is not a blame game, either apportioning blame or accepting blame.

Disclosure is a meaningful process and a journey about learning. It is about truth, accountability and professionalism. A woman having experienced an adverse outcome on her journey shared her story, emphasizing 'you hold our lives in your hands and we want to hold you in high regard' (Murphy, 2013). A culture of honesty, openness and transparency including apologizing and explaining what happened (NPSA, 2009) is crucial to facilitate open disclosure.

Each person benefits from kind, respectful introductions such as 'hello my name is' followed by refreshingly honest, open and transparent communication; this should be the norm. Giving and receiving an explanation and an apology facilitates healing for everyone. Only then can forgiveness, recovery and learning take root. Better maternity care can only be achieved if blame is abandoned as a measuring tool. Our shared primary goal of high-quality maternity care is achievable only when transparency, fairness, compassion and always kindness are deemed essential for all.

KEY MESSAGES

- Open disclosure needs 'buy in' from senior managers and strong leadership is paramount.
- The main barriers to the open disclosure process are fear of litigation and reputational damage; therefore protective legislation is required to facilitate clinicians to confidently apologize and fully disclose to service users and their families.
- Staff involved in adverse events are often referred to as the 'second victim' so it is crucial that staff are also cared for and supported following the adverse event.
- In the immediate aftermath of an adverse event it can be difficult to de-

termine what went wrong. At this point the service user/family should be informed of the known facts at the time. Hearsay and speculation should be avoided as this can lead to confusion and heightened anxiety.

- There needs to be appropriate follow-up support for service users and their families following an adverse event to promote confidence and reassurance in relation to their ongoing care.
- The healthcare organization's support must be visible to patients and staff, including communicating to the media.

ACTION POINTS

- Be open and honest about your actions.
- Remember the power of a respectful introduction, to everyone.
- 'Being prepared' prior to holding an open disclosure meeting(s) is key and influences the success of the process.
- Integrate open disclosure into patient safety initiatives, applicable policies, procedures and standards.

25 They don't know what they don't know

Amali Lokugamage and Theresa Bourne

Professor Murray Enkin, who co-authored the influential Guide to Effective Care in Pregnancy and Childbirth *(Enkin et al, 2000), which was a
precursor to the development of the Cochrane Collaboration, referred to the
concept of doctors 'not knowing what they didn't know' in a guest editorial
in the journal* Birth *(Enkin, 2008). His paper described the assimilation of
knowledge through medical education. It dealt with what he termed 'The
Seven Stages of Ignorance', ranging from the First Stage: Innocence. You
Know You Don't Know, But You're Sure You Can Learn; to the Seventh
Stage: Ignorance. You Know That You Don't Know, Others Know That You
Don't Know, and It Doesn't Matter! In the course of the paper, he suggested
that medical students and doctors assume that their medical syllabus deliv-
ers all the knowledge and skills that they need to know to become experts in
maternity care. This is despite the fact that there is very little in the area of
humanities, not withstanding the strongly social nature of maternity care
provision. This chapter explores some of the implications of omitting social-
ly relevant knowledge and learning from the basic training of obstetricians.
It presents a new approach that is designed to fill the gap, and, in the process, to alert student doctors to the need for a humanized approach to the
maternity care they provide in the future. The aim is to consider the impact
of standard medical education, and of alternative approaches, on the delivery of kindness, dignity and respect to women within maternity care. In doing so it recognizes that the medical student will qualify as a doctor and the
knowledge and skills that they develop during their training will influence
the way they practise and provide care after qualification.*

The impact of normative assumptions about medical guidelines

In an exercise undertaken by one of us (AL) with medical students, they
are asked what percentage of the total obstetrics and gynaecology clinical guidelines are made from high-quality evidence. There is a general assumption that at least 80% of guidelines are drawn from grade A
(the most unbiased and reliable) evidence. However, an evaluation of the
American College of Obstetricians and Gynecologists' (ACOG) clinical
guidelines revealed that only one third of the recommendations put forth
by the College in its practice bulletins are based on good and consistent
scientific evidence (Wright *et al*, 2011). A similar analysis of the UK Royal College of Obstetricians and Gynaecologists' guidelines showed that

only 9-12% of the recommendations are from grade A evidence (Prusova *et al*, 2014). Block (2007) argues strongly that much of what is advised in relation to patient safety, often to the determent of maternal choice, is not founded in rigorous research.

The popular misconception within medicine that guidelines are robust indicators of best practice potentially results in the belief that evidence-based medicine (EBM) is a rule to be followed for all members of a population, when it actually refers to the application of the best available evidence to inform clinical care in each individual case (Sackett, 1996). This is reinforced with the use of some clinical models (Haynes *et al*, 2002), but, generally, in practice, this misconception leads to little consideration of patient choice, and a resistance to individualizing care to suit the patient. Trisha Greenhalgh (2012) is a strong critic of evidence-based medicine (EBM) and has a special interest in the philosophical aspects of medical care, and in particular the tension between 'rational' scientific evidence and the messy practicalities of real-world medicine and policy-making. Greenhalgh is concerned with the limitations of the fundamentally linear and reductionist paradigm of EBM, when it meets the highly complex and relentlessly contextual problems encountered in the clinic, at the bedside, and around the policy-making table. She has founded a #realEBM movement on the social media platform Twitter to overturn such prevalent attitudes.

Paucity of information on biobehavioural aspects of birth

Birth and pregnancy lay down many of the factors that have implications for societal health in the longer term (Lokugamage, 2011). The opportunity to explore the sociology and physiology that underpins these longer-term outcomes is vital to fully understand the implications of practising in certain ways as a doctor. Being present at a spontaneous physiological birth reinforces this knowledge. Despite curricula changes to reflect the social and attitudinal aspects of care alongside clinical knowledge (RCOG, 2009), the growing numbers of students, in the UK at least, means that the feasibility of being present for a meaningful length of time during normal birth is limited (Lumsden and Symonds, 2010). This is further hampered by the increasing rate of birth interventions, including the high caesarean rates and labour induction (Health and Social Information Centre, 2013), which means that, even when students are able to accompany a labouring woman, they are unlikely to observe the physiological and biobehavioural aspects of a spontaneous birth (Stone, 2012).

Midwifery-led continuity models of care and case-loading are associated with a reduction in caesareans and intervention rates in birth (Health and Social Information Centre, 2013; Sandall *et al*, 2013; Tracey *et al*, 2013) However, not all curricula offer medical students placements with midwives, and especially not in environments such as home or birth centres, where more spontaneous vaginal birth is more likely to occur (Lumsden and Symonds, 2010).

Learning to cope with uncertainty

There appears an innate perception that birth is an event waiting to go wrong. Medical education has a strong focus on ill health and repair or healing but birth falls outside this remit for most women (Lokugamage, 2011). The emphasis on potential ill health has a tendency to create anxiety, not only in the parents but also in the health professionals caring for them. Decisions made based on this philosophy impact on natural biophysical events, and impede normal physiology, changing the course and outcomes of labour and birth. Actions may be taken to prevent potential harm for the few, which end up causing actual harm for the many (Block, 2007). This may have much wider consequences for the mother and baby and their future health, including physiological, psychological, emotional, sexual and societal impacts. Teaching about these lasting consequences is not usually evident within the curriculum.

Developing resilience in the context of uncertainty is a learnt skill, which may be resisted in healthcare. There is more about resilience in midwifery in this book, but, in general, actions in maternity care are designed to rule out risk through attempts to manage and control events (Page and Mander, 2014). As fewer health professionals are willing to work with uncertainty, capacity in this area is diminishing, thus perpetuating the problem.

Medical education in healthcare human rights

In England, the new undergraduate syllabus at University College London medical school contains education about healthcare human rights, and the rights of patients, children and those with disabilities are underlined in the medical school curriculum (RCOG, 2009).

However, in terms of postgraduate education for obstetricians, the RCOG has only recently become formally involved in postgraduate multidisciplinary training in reproductive human rights. The 2014 celebration of International Women's Day was devoted to this issue, and a recommendation has been made that the RCOG/FIGO (International Federation of Gynecology and Obstetrics) human rights checklist should be used in clinical training. The RCOG Vice President, Professor Lesley

Regan (2014) has broadcast a video stating that the 'importance of incorporating an understanding of human rights into women's healthcare is that there is now good evidence to demonstrate that when clinicians of all sorts of denominations (doctors, nurses, midwives, healthcare assistants) understand the importance of protecting and preserving human rights, the quality of care is so much better for patients' (vimeo.com/92744531). She comments that this issue is as vital for the UK as it is for developing countries.

The exercise of human rights requires a shift in power to the user rather than the caregiver to improve autonomy in decision making, through approaches such as what Lowe terms 'subtle cohesion' (Lowe, 2013, p138). Whilst acknowledging that there are a few clients who may be uncomfortable with the responsibility that comes with an increase in autonomy, Patel (2013) notes that the main issue is that many health professionals lack the training to support this change.

Economic drivers of medicine

As for most other medical disciplines, obstetrics has become more target driven (Lumsden and Symonds, 2010). This can mean less time in individual clinical consultations, leading to a concentration on the immediate issue rather than healthcare in its fullest sense. This lack of patient centredness can limit knowledge based on a full understanding of the issues that are important to the health of the individual, and the specific implications for that client, and can be associated with disrespectful or even abusive behaviour (Francis, 2013; Newdick and Banbury, 2013). Further, Lowe (2014) claims that standardization of healthcare does not always lead to efficiency or even effective care as it misses vital clues that are indivually relevant and informative, but that may not be measured with standard tools and checklists.

Symon (2006) identifies that risk and choice are not always paradoxical, as activity can be undertaken where risk is understood and accepted when the focus is on risk awareness rather than aversion. He highlights that a lot of medical training occurs in acute settings where alternatives and time may be limited and where decisions and choices are 'doctor-led' because there is not enough opportunity for proper discussion with the patient/service user. This has an obvious impact when working in an area where the decisions are made by women using the maternity service. The problem is compounded if the student or doctor lacks knowledge of physiological birth, limiting the information they can share when facilitating decision making.

Teaching medical students about staff attitudes to women

Childbearing women have heightened senses during pregnancy, labour and birth, and many women recall small details years after the event. It is, therefore, not surprising that staff attitudes and relationships are what women raise as a major issue during and following birth (Baker *et al*, 2005). With the pressures of targets and the inadequate opportunities within practice the medical student is limited in gaining full experience in this area. University College London is attempting to address this with the use of patient pathways, allowing students to share some of the journey and recognize the elements that women themselves identify as important in maternity care.

Conclusion

Best practice is not just a learnt process from the classroom environment. It is developed and built from what a student witnesses within practice. The language we use with women is often mechanistic as well as alien to the woman, and it works to ensure that control remains with the health practitioner (Kitzinger, 2005). Furthermore, the manner of our care can deteriorate insidiously without awareness (Aronson, 2013), perhaps driven by the pressures of time, and we can become embedded in the healthcare culture. Additionally, pressure of work and the critical incidents we meet may impact on our role and how we both communicate and interact with our future clients (de Boer *et al*, 2011). Mechanisms to address this include personal reflection, group discussion and clinical supervision. However, utilizing the data collected on the client experience and listening to women is the first major step in recognizing where improvements need to be made (Coulter *et al*, 2014). This could be integrated into the medical student curriculum to strengthen these aspects within future care. Lewis (2013) warns that health system reactions that result in increased surveillance or risk avoidance have missed the point and that a service that listens and attends to the needs of women is more likely to bring a sustainable change within the delivery of healthcare. Teaching our medical students and obstetricians about the nature and consequences of physiological labour and birth, and about what women think, believe, feel and value about childbirth, is an important step in increasing skilled, knowledgeable, compassionate obstetrics in future practice.

KEY MESSAGES

- Students will not see kindness, dignity and respect unless they have the opportunity to witness it and see it modelled within the care of women and their families.

- The opportunity to meet with women to discuss care, exploring aspects of how kindness, dignity and respect were demonstrated within that care (or not), is an important tool for learning. This should be followed with a structured space to reflect and underpin the development of these qualities in care.
- The medical curriculum needs to provide knowledge and skills beyond the purely physical features of care. The attention to the biosocial aspects provides the opportunity to consider how kindness, dignity and respect can be incorporated into care as well as improve birth outcomes.
- The integration of human rights throughout care, with a clear understanding of autonomy and how the health professional can impact on this, is vital within medical education.

ACTION POINTS

- Teaching and clinical staff should ensure that the opportunity to engage and participate in the care of women and their families during normal labour and birth is available for medical students and qualified doctors. Those designing medical education curricula should ensure that the biopsychosocial aspects of the birth experience and the implications for immediate, long-term and societal health are included in teaching sessions.
- All medical students and postgraduate doctors should be taught that human rights are an issue even in the UK. They should be made fully aware that autonomy is not an optional extra, but an essential element in client decision making.
- Meaningful opportunities to listen to women and their needs within the childbirth continuum should be provided within the medical curriculum.
- Health professionals need to model compassionate, respectful and effective care to students and trainee doctors working with women in developing health professionals and a service for the future.

26 With-woman, with-student: developing a woman and family-centred midwifery recruitment strategy and curriculum for caring

Anna Byrom, Shelagh Heneghan and Mercedes Perez-Bottella

This chapter outlines how we facilitate the identification and development of kindness, compassion, sensitivity and mutual respect within student midwives. We consider the application of salutogenesis theory to midwifery recruitment and education practice, and include a review of our student selection strategy and our case-based learning curriculum.

Beginning at the end

'What will the midwife of the future be expected and be able to do?' 'What kind of midwifery practitioner is needed and desired in the 21st century?' 'What sort of midwife do women and their families really want?'

These are the questions we asked as we set out to update our midwifery curriculum and recruitment process at the University of Central Lancashire, in the North-West of England in 2012. There are many perspectives to be considered when planning and implementing a pre-registration midwifery curriculum design and recruitment strategy, ranging from the Government, the professional body for nursing and midwifery (the Nursing and Midwifery Council – NMC), the Royal College of Midwives (RCM), educationalists, academics, managers and researchers to clinicians, students, auditors, the World Health Organization (WHO) and commissioners of maternity services (Department of Health [DoH], 2010, 2010a; Kings Fund 2011, 2012; NMC 2008, 2009, 2011, 2012). But the most important perspective of all is that of the woman who engages with the maternity services generally and with midwifery care in particular, as she travels through her pregnancy, birth and parenthood journey. Careful consideration of all these factors enabled us to canvas a broad range of desirable characteristics of the 'ideal' midwife. These are captured in the figure on page 172 as an overview.

With the woman and her family as our focus we set out to develop a recruitment strategy and midwifery curriculum that would meet the needs of the many and varied stakeholders in midwife preparation, but especially those of childbearing women and their families who, for several years, have stated that kindness, compassion, sensitivity and mutual respect have been lost in the technocentric, risk-obsessed culture that has evolved in maternity care (DoH, 2012a).

This chapter outlines how we facilitate the identification and development of kindness, compassion, sensitivity and mutual respect within student midwives. We consider the application of salutogenesis theory to midwifery recruitment and education practice; to include a review of our student selection strategy and our case-based learning curriculum (Antonovsky, 1979; Mezirow, 1991; Rogoff, 1999; Kim *et al*, 2006).

A salutogenic approach: through a positive lens

In recognition of women globally as individuals and of the childbearing continuum as a journey that can be considered on a spectrum from smooth and uneventful to complex and challenging, our recruitment and curriculum philosophy was underpinned by a salutogenic orientation to healthcare (Antonovsky, 1979, 1993). As summarised in Table 1, salutogenesis represents an approach that moves away from the traditional pathological paradigm of dichotomizing normal/abnormal and low-risk/high-risk to perceiving health on a transient continuum situated within the context of our environment and social lives (Linstrom and Eriksson, 2010). It is a philosophical position well-aligned with traditional midwifery approaches which embraces being 'with-woman' and understanding childbearing as a healthy physical and psychosocial phenomenon.

The recruitment strategy and the curriculum have been designed to ensure student midwives' learning, skill development and care delivery are focused on the promotion of health and wellbeing irrespective of the classification of risk assigned to the childbearing woman, baby or family and that both education and practice are sensitive to the socio-cultural context of all individuals concerned. The socio-cultural context includes students and their teachers as well as pregnant women and their families as they learn with and from each other, and develop their sense of coherence (Antonovsky, 1979) during their respective journeys. Before we examine how salutogenesis influences our curriculum design and delivery it is useful to consider how it underpins our recruitment strategy.

Finding compassion – shifting the focus of our recruitment process

Why change?

Courage, commitment and compassion can be learnt through education and role modelling but these are qualities that individuals possess to a greater or lesser degree in an almost innate manner (Trinh and Edge, 2012). In order to successfully generate a midwifery workforce that displays those values, a major factor is identifying at the point of entry into midwifery education those individuals who already display those qualities.

Table 1: Salutogenesis theory

Salutogenesis theory was first introduced by Aaron Antonovsky (1979). The term can be translated as 'the origin of health' in which the main premise is to look for what contributes to the creation of health rather than pursuing the traditional enquiry paradigm which searches for the cause of disease within a pathogenic framework focused on risk aversion and risk prevention (Beck, 1992; Giddens, 1990; McKenzie Bryers and van Teijlingen, 2010).

In a revolutionary new view of the health/disease dichotomy, the theory proposed health as a continuum between 'total health and total unhealth' (Lindstrom and Eriksson, 2010). Individuals could be placed at any time on any part of this continuum and their attempts would always be focused on moving towards the health end of the continuum.

He conceptualized this construct in what he called the sense of coherence (SOC) which is central to the salutogenesis theory and incorporates the elements of manageability, comprehensibility and meaningfulness. Central to his theory was also the term General Resistance Resources, which provide the prerequisites for the development of the SOC (Eriksson, 2007). They refer to the skills individuals have to combat the stressors in life, including people's own capacities but also their ability to access resources in their immediate environment (money, self-esteem, social relations, beliefs) (Lindstrom and Eriksson, 2006).

However, the key lies not only in having access to the resources, but also being able to use them in a healthy promoting way. Thus a balance can be accomplished between the extent of the stressors and the abilities of individuals to utilize all available resources (Lindsom and Eriksson, 2010). Since disease, unpredictability and chaos are natural parts of everyday life, he concluded that people who managed to integrate these concepts within their assimilation of the world would be much better suited to play down their importance and live lives closer to the health end of the continuum.

For more information please visit the salutogenesis website: salutogenesis.hv.se

---

Traditional interviews can fail to recognize those individuals who have a genuine caring nature. As such our current recruitment process for the BSc (Hons) midwifery programme has undergone important changes. We have moved from a single individual interview approach to a Multi Mini Interview (MMI) day. This provides a better platform for candidates to show the qualities and attributes they possess to become a competent midwife as described by the NMC (2009), and in line with the Compassion in Practice document (DoH, 2012). This was also intended to allow the recruitment team to make better informed choices about the candidates recruited.

What changed?

Our new process, employing an MMI approach (MSC Medical, 2012), consists of a series of interactive stations where candidates are presented with scenarios that they have to respond to. These scenarios have been devised to test the candidates' abilities relating to the '6Cs': care, compassion, competence, courage, commitment and communication. Competence is tested via multiple choice questions around midwifery/ maternity care. There is a growing body of evidence that shows that MMIs are a more sensitive and effective method than the traditional interview in identifying those personal attributes required from the student (Salvatori 2001; Eva, Rosenfeld, Reiter and Norman, 2004).

The use of scenarios during the MMIs helps candidates to explore responses, reactions and emotions and encourages them to think about how they would behave, care or manage the situations presented and why. It has been positively evaluated by candidates to date. The use of scenarios or cases also aligns well to the case-based learning design chosen for our curriculum model. The following section will offer insight into the development, design and delivery of our salutogenesis-informed, case-based learning approach to midwifery education.

Student-centredness for woman-centred care – a review of our case-based learning curriculum

Linking theory with education practice

With salutogenesis as our guiding curriculum philosophy, we looked to education theory to identify an appropriate curriculum model. It was essential that our curriculum reflected the standards expected by the United Kingdom (UK) NMC and the key priorities outlined in our stakeholder meetings, attended by midwives, leaders, researchers and service-users (NMC, 2009). To keep these principles at the heart of our curriculum development we developed core themes to be covered by the curriculum – see diagram below.

More importantly, however, our aim was to design a curriculum that would enable student midwives to facilitate caring with compassion and kindness for childbearing women and their families. It is well established that the key to enabling effective compassionate midwifery care is to locate the woman and her family at the centre of the service provision and through the development of a loving, responsive and nurturing midwife-mother relationship (Kirkham, 2010). Utilizing the concepts of

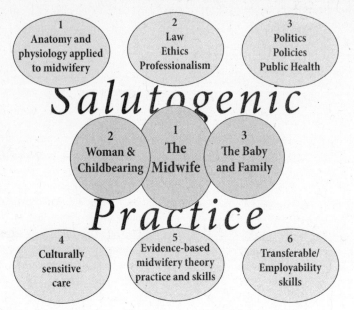

Figure: Curriculum themes developed in our stakeholder meetings

woman-centred and family-centred care, underpinned by salutogenesis, we turned to case-based learning as an appropriate curriculum model that offered a structure to ensure women and families remained the focus of our midwifery education delivery.

Why CBL?
Exploring specific, realistic, case studies is well aligned to salutogenesis theory. Students are encouraged to locate individuals within the context of physical, psychosocial and cultural influencing factors with a focus on how the midwife might work to enhance individuals' sense of coherence through improved manageability, comprehensibility and meaningfulness. Case-based learning (CBL) offers a move away from definition-based learning and, more importantly, away from modularized fragmented health education that presents physiology separately from sociology, ecology and psychology. CBL is andragogical (adult teaching/learning) and poses contextualized questions that are based upon clinical or non-clinical 'real life' cases. These cases are developed to encourage students to use enquiry methods, stimulating and underpinning the acquisition of knowledge, skills and appropriate professional attitudes and behaviours (Williams, 2005). Crucially CBL is a participatory education method that

stimulates students to become engaged in their own and others' learning, building on prior experiences and supporting the development of life-long learners; perfect for midwifery education.

Importantly, CBL enabled our six curriculum themes, identified as essential during our stakeholder curriculum development meetings, to be integrated into students' daily learning across all facets of the curriculum. The following section will outline how we organized and delivered the curriculum.

Engaging with CBL – the practicalities

As a midwifery team we worked together to develop the CBL content and delivery structure. Team work was essential for successful case development and delivery. In the development phase it felt resource intensive, as we required whole-team input for individual sessions. As we have become experienced with both case development and facilitation we have now ensured workload is shared effectively across the team and case-leads now take feedback from all groups; reducing the need for multiple facilitators.

Students are organized into small groups of four or five to engage with our CBL curriculum. Group membership is rotated each theory block to support student relationship growth across the cohort. Small group work helps to increase student engagement, improve confidence during group feedback and encourages effective group management. Importantly, small group working strengthens students' team work, reflection and communication skills – essential for midwifery practice and compassionate care. It is an element of CBL that enables students to enhance their employability through the development of core skills.

Student engagement with the curriculum follows a clear process to ensure consistency and quality across cases and between case leads/facilitators. This is an essential feature of curriculum development. Having a simple and structured framework for each case, or aspect of a case, enabled students to assimilate with a new approach to learning. Regular communication, evaluation and feedback between facilitators, students and course leaders ensured the course content and cases were adapted, reviewed and revised to respond to individual, group and class needs. The responsive capacity of CBL has been an overwhelming benefit. It has enabled us to care for students' needs and to respond to our own needs as midwifery educators. This in turn gives the student time to focus on their own learning.

Initial evaluation - challenges and success

The whole-curriculum shift to CBL has been a steep learning curve for the teaching team and students alike. We all felt a sense of moving out of our comfort zone. As educators there was a concern that leaving students to learn for themselves may affect achievement of the learning outcomes for the course. This was accompanied by apprehension that our role as teacher was in some way diminished – that we offered a reduced service with CBL due to less formal teaching. Indeed this sentiment has been provoked at times with a few students offering feedback that CBL makes it a 'do-it-yourself' course. However as we have come to the end of our first year engaging with the curriculum for both the three-year and shortened 20-month BSc midwifery degrees we feel confident that our course is appropriately 'do-it-yourself'. When we reflect on our original vision for the course which was to 'develop compassionate midwives who are life-long, motivated learners; prepared to drive the profession forward for women, babies and families' we are reminded how appropriate CBL has been. CBL ensures consistent engagement, learning and development for individual students. Our new role as facilitators of learning has encouraged a new approach to support and leadership. We are with-student every step of their journey offering individual feedback that is no longer restricted to the end of a module or the end of year, but given after every case feedback at least every week. We follow the students as they navigate the childbearing woman's journey – hand-in-hand exploring changes in physiology, impacts of psychosocial wellbeing and challenges for maternity services and the midwifery profession. From day one students are researchers, team members, and care-makers for the woman and family. As their teachers we echo the work of the midwife – work that is beautifully described by Lao Tzu in the *Tao Te Ching*:

> *The wise leader does not intervene unnecessarily.*
>
> *The leader's presence is felt, but often the group runs itself.*
>
> *Remember you are facilitating another person's process. It is not your process.*
>
> *Do not intrude. Do not control. Do not force your own needs and insights in to the foreground. If you do not trust a person's process, that person will not trust you.*
>
> *Imagine that you are a midwife; you are assisting at someone else's birth. Do good without show or fuss. Facilitate what is happening rather than what you think ought to be happening.*
>
> *If you must take the lead, lead so that the mother is helped, yet still free and in charge.*
>
> *When the baby is born, the mother will rightly say – 'we did it ourselves'*
>
> *(Dreher, 1996)*

This is our reminder about the nature of our role as facilitators of our CBL curriculum. We are also encouraged by overwhelmingly positive student feedback.

Looking to the future – our conclusions and recommendations

In addition to enabling a shift in focus from disease to health and wellbeing, salutogenesis also offers an approach to selecting, supporting and nurturing student midwives. It encourages us, as midwifery educators, to consider ways to review and support potential, new and existing students' sense of coherence as we guide them to develop skills to support childbearing women and families to develop theirs. Salutogenesis is simultaneously a philosophy to inform learning strategies and pastoral mentoring approaches for individual students. It offers a theoretical underpinning of our objectives to support the development of midwives who are capable of successful change implementation in those scientific-bureaucratic healthcare systems that prevent practitioners from being with woman/woman centred.

We believe that our curriculum is a compassionate curriculum and, as such, prepares students to 'be' compassionate. We model, through our responsive and nurturing approach to learning facilitation, how to be a compassionate midwife. Guided by salutogenesis we work to enhance students' sense of coherence – by placing them at the centre of their learning experience, and in doing so demonstrate an approach they can adopt to support the childbearing woman and her family. We promote woman-centred care through our student-centred curriculum; 'being' what we hope our students will become – compassionate midwives of the future.

KEY MESSAGES

- Salutogenesis is a philosophical framework for midwifery recruitment and curriculum development.
- Look for candidates who demonstrate possession of the 6Cs during recruitment by using role play and life-focused scenarios.
- Use a student-centred curriculum aimed at enhancing woman-centred care.
- Case-based learning creates midwives for the future – responsive, caring, reflective and competent.

ACTION POINTS

- Start with an agreed philosophy and a clear vision of who you want the midwife to be as a result of your training.

- Foster a culture of team work through regular meetings, away days and staff-student team-building events.
- A cohort lead is vital to ensure consistency across all aspects of the curriculum.
- Support each other through the challenges by sharing ideas, resources and experiences.
- Ask each student cohort to evaluate their learning and experiences regularly. It's important to highlight positive achievements with each other and students.

27 Care and compassion count: supporting student midwives in practice

Carmel McCalmont and Sue Lees

Most healthcare workers enter their profession with a desire to provide compassionate care (Youngson, 2012). However, recent reports have highlighted that care in the National Health Service has not always met the needs of service users and subsequently there has been an increased focus on the importance of kindness and compassion. The Chief Nursing Officer's vision (CBCNO/DoH, 2012) is encapsulated in the document Compassion in Practice which identifies the '6Cs': care, compassion, competence, communication, courage and commitment. Health Education England is currently undertaking work on 'personalised maternity care' reflecting the philosophy of the 6Cs and recognizing that feedback from women is an important aspect of a practitioner's development.

Education plays a vital role in the preparation of effective practitioners who are both technically skilled and exhibit the 6Cs. In order to develop and internalize these professional values, students need to be treated with kindness and compassion and learn to apply them in the care that they provide. This chapter will explore the development and use of a Check and Challenge proforma through which professional values may be explored with students.

The nature of the UK student midwife programme

The Nursing and Midwifery Council (NMC) requires that students spend at least forty per cent of the programme in clinical practice (NMC, 2008), working with women and families under the supervision of a midwife mentor, with the remainder of the time being spent in a higher education institution. Effective mentorship during the clinical component is essential; student midwives learn through observing the mentor as she interacts with women and families (Hall, 2013). Students note that a good mentor is approachable and a positive role model who influences their practice (Hughes and Fraser, 2010). As Robin Youngerson has said, 'Compassion is portrayed in the smallest acts' (Youngson, 2012) and a mentor who addresses the 'little things' can influence a student who is trying to determine the type of practitioner she or he would like to be upon registration.

Throughout the midwifery programme, students have the opportunity to provide feedback and report their perception of care. They may do this within the clinical setting and/or within the higher education institution through, for example, module and course evaluations. Sometimes the silence… has been deafening (Peate, 2012). In order to empower students to be open, the Check and Challenge process was developed, with the use of a carefully designed proforma.

Development and impact of Check and Challenge

The idea was generated in October 2012 following a student evaluation event. It was recognized that, although the Head of Midwifery (HoM) of the maternity unit spoke with students on a daily basis about their experience, which they reported was positive, a different perspective was aired at the evaluation event. Anecdotally, students reported that they did not wish to raise issues with the HoM as they might wish to apply for a job in her team at the end of the programme. The comments were acted upon, and a form was developed, tested with one cohort of students and refined so that rich information was obtained.

Although the proforma explores student experience, mentorship, statutory supervision and the woman's experience, it also potentially enables a fruitful relationship between the HoM and each student. The exercise aims to ensure that the student feels valued, and a true member of the team rather than being just 'the student'. Because students have to obtain feedback from the women they care for, the exercise enables the HoM to discuss the care that women and families have received. At the point of registration, competition for posts is high so feedback from families adds another dimension upon which the student may build.

The HoM has been able to interact with students and has found that they highlight personal and academic pressures during the protected time they have together. This has enabled the HoM, and the education team, to strengthen the support available to student midwives and has increased the partnership working between practice and higher education.

The strength of this process was tested in September 2013 when, at the course evaluation event that followed introduction of the new system, feedback from the students was consistent with the information collected through the Check and Challenge proforma during the year. Students reported that issues were resolved in a timely manner. The Check and Challenge proforma was commended as good practice by the NMC at a programme approval event in 2013. At the course evaluation event in September 2014, students commented that 'lecturers take the time to get to know us as individuals' and specifically highlighted Check and Challenge as one of the strengths of the clinical component of the programme, which made them feel *valued and supported by the Head of Midwifery*.

Hearing students' voices

The following quotes illustrate the kind of responses that have been associated with the introduction of the Check and Challenge system:

> 'In my first year I didn't feel valued: people used to call for the student. I was a number, not a person. When Check and Challenge began, because the HoM knew my name, everyone started calling me by name. I feel much more like a member of the team now.'

> 'I really did not appreciate how close education and practice are. My named tutor knew that I had been involved in an obstetric emergency, which had scared me. The HoM came to see me after the emergency and we did a Check and Challenge. She was kind to me, we had a debrief and I felt much better. When I told my tutor she already knew about the event so it made it easier to discuss.'

> 'On my second placement my mentorship was a bit all over the place. I was with different people every day so I didn't get my objectives discussed early. I didn't want to say but at my Check and Challenge I was assured that it needed to be put right for my future. It was and I would not be worried to say again.'

> 'My mentor is great. She teaches me so well and supports me at work. She is such a good midwife. I am lucky to have her. I love my training.'

> 'How would you access a Supervisor of Midwives? – I would phone switch board or ask the co-ordinator.'

> 'Did you know who your mentor was before you started your placement? – Yes I knew her name. Have you worked most of your shifts with her? Yes all of them. I have been really lucky we get on very well.'

Conclusion

The extracts from the Check and Challenge proforma and discussions with the students demonstrate how spending a short time investing in directed conversation can have a positive impact on them. Kindness and compassion towards trainees will hopefully ensure that they will learn from that and embed it in their practice. Check and Challenge is a very simple way of making people feel valued.

KEY MESSAGES

- Most practitioners enter their profession with a desire to provide compassionate care.
- Effective mentorship is crucial to the development of a caring, compassionate practitioner.
- Students learn through observation and role modelling.

- Kindness and compassion are key and must be reaffirmed as core values in maternity care.

ACTION POINTS

- As a qualified member of staff, make sure that you get to know the students you encounter.
- All Heads of Midwifery should ensure they are visible and accessible so that students feel able to discuss practice.
- Consider introducing something like the Check and Challenge system to ensure that students' views and experiences are taken into account.

28 Compassionate care, midwives, women and forum theatre: two tales from practice

Adele Stanley, Gemma Boyd, Anna Byrom and Kirsten Baker

This chapter includes reflections of our experiences working as midwife actors with Progress Theatre. We share our personal experiences of using theatre methods to explore midwifery and wider healthcare practice. These offer accounts of related organizational and personal influences and how they impact on care provision in maternity services. We aim to demonstrate how theatre can be used to unpack life experiences, and how it can stimulate maternity care practitioners to reflect on their personal responses to their work experiences. As such we provide examples of the theatre techniques we use to explore cultures, beliefs and behaviours in practice against the backdrop of organizational context and constraints.

A forum introduction: Progress Theatre background

Formed in 1999, Progress Theatre is a group of midwives from a range of clinical and educational settings who also have a background in theatre and drama. The work we do is based on the emancipatory approach of the South American dramaturge Augusto Boal. This approach encourages a shared platform between participants and players – a space where both the members of the theatre company and those they are performing to can examine life together. By placing the spectator (audience) at the centre of the working piece Boal's theatre methods aim to represent different aspects of reality creating the possibility to consider varying solutions and change. Using Boal's forum theatre methods we explore issues relating to healthcare and maternity services with an audience of midwives and health professionals. Forum theatre encourages the audience to interact with the performance, at times pausing the action to offer suggestions, ideas and ways to 'be' different. Table 1 offers some forum theatre methods that can be applied to a range of education contexts.

We have devised and performed shows on complex and emerging aspects of professional culture including workplace bullying, sexual abuse and maternity care, and the impact of the risk culture on clinical care. We have explored the tensions and rewards of interagency working with shows about domestic violence and drug abuse in a number of multidisciplinary fora. Workshop material and techniques can be adapted to capture key learning points in forms other than a half-day workshop.

Table 1: Forum theatre methods

With the examples included below it is useful for someone to become what Boal calls a 'joker' or facilitator between the actors and participants/spectators.

Forum method	Description	Application
Network image	Participants use their bodies to create a physical representation or image of their experiences. This can be a static 'photo-shot' image or a moving production based on audience-led suggestions associated with the topic under consideration. *Aim*: to explore shared experiences.	*Example* Explore the pressures experienced by 'every midwife'. A participant stands on the stage, representing 'every midwife'. All participants are invited to suggest all the things that might impact on 'every midwife'. Suggestions might include: Workload, Paperwork, Colleagues Students, Audits, Home-life, etc These are then represented physically by asking members of the audience to play out each suggestion and show physically how these might impact on the midwife. For example: • Workload might press on her/his shoulders • Students might pull her/his arm You are then left with a physical image of the pressures midwives might face – this allows the participants to consider their own and others' experiences.
Stop think	Participants watch a scene and are given the forum to clap and stop the action at any point to say, in the first person, what they think the characters are thinking and feeling. *Aim*: to consider other peoples' perspectives and develop empathy.	*Example* Act out a role play from any practice scenario eg, a busy hospital environment. As the scene unfolds encourage participants to clap to pause the performance. Ask them to say, in the first person, what each character is thinking and/or feeling. Try and encourage the participants to stay focused on what the character thinks and feels and why rather than what they think and feel.

Forum method	Description	Application
'Others' shoes'	Participants become 'spect-actors' and get involved with the action of the theatre by stopping the action and suggesting changes. They are encouraged to take the part of the actor and try out their suggestions. *Aim*: to experience things from other peoples' perspectives and try out solutions for practice.	*Example* Act out a scene that identifies some of the relational challenges commonly found in midwifery practice. Participants are then invited to stop the action by clapping their hands – they can then ask one of the midwives in the scene to change their behaviour, offering practical suggestions to the actor or trying the suggestions out themselves and becoming part of the performance.

Examples include keynote presentations at conferences as well as scaled-down, hour-long presentations as part of a teaching and learning event.

We begin our workshops with a vivid research-based portrayal of the issue under exploration. This provides participants with a springboard for a participatory workshop in which we use established techniques for engaging individuals in a searching consideration of their own and others' practice. We then use a range of forum theatre methods such as 'stop think' and 'network image' (see *Table 1* for details); these help participants to examine organizational culture or personal responses and behaviour. Participants have commented that engagement with the activities of our workshops stimulates them to see things differently, that they feel enabled to change their own practice positively, and that they have gained new and valuable insights on seemingly intractable problems.

Endorsements for our work have come from a wide spectrum of practitioners: clinical leads and supervisors, practitioners, authors, researchers, educators and students. The vivid engagement that can be evoked by this form of teaching and learning is due in part to the fact that those portraying the events in each scenario – as midwife actors – have personally lived through such events, or something very like them, in their working lives. Good preparation in researching the experiences of stakeholders is also vital, along with the adoption of an iterative approach where the insights of the stakeholders can be fed back into the process of devising the specific play under development.

Being part of Progress Theatre as midwife actors we are afforded unique opportunities to listen, share and learn from a wide range of midwives and other practitioners during the interactive workshops we deliver. These experiences have helped us to develop our own approach to midwifery and working within maternity services across the United Kingdom. The following offers personal accounts, from two of our midwife actors, exploring the impact of working with Progress Theatre.

Whose shoes are they anyway? Adele's reflections on Progress

Compassionate care encompasses empathy, kindness, and trust. Progress Theatre are interested in exploring channels of communication in maternity care using interactive forum theatre methods to encourage participants to 'walk in each others' shoes'. This enables participants to examine different perspectives and challenging situations whilst 'playing' with alternative ideas and ways of working. The hope is that these explorations encourage empathy and influence positive practice outcomes.

Using theatre methods to actively engage with 'real-life' scenarios and situations inevitably involves vicariously experiencing the pain of lack of compassion but also the warmth of being in a kind and supportive environment, as part of the immersion in the acting moment. For example, in a workshop, devised with student midwives, we show a scenario wherein a positive situation between a student midwife and a labouring woman changes into a much darker one when there is a sudden emergency. The student is pushed out of the picture because of the emergency situation. She is left feeling incompetent, anxious and guilty because she has left the birthing woman's side. The woman is denied the security of the student's kind and supportive care. Their trustful relationship is shattered and nothing positive is coming out of this situation except a live baby. After the play has been shown once, the audience are asked if one of them would like to come and take the place of any of the actors, to change the behaviours they have witnessed. The audience member who takes on the role of the student must find ways of enacting the scene differently using only the student's language and behaviour to reach a different outcome. The process allows the audience member (and those witnessing the drama) to feel the student's anxiety which is a much more powerful experience than being told to do something differently. Working as one of the midwife actors with Progress Theatre, hearing and feeling how others experience situations, encourages personal learning and development. Now, when working clinically as a senior midwife, in any emergency situation I will always find a useful role for the student and work to include her in the real-life drama of everyday practice.

Sharing our baggage – easing the load

Progress Theatre have devised work on subjects as varied as domestic abuse, substance misuse, bullying and sexual abuse. What they all have in common is the sense of the invisible baggage a person can bring into any given situation and how that experience can be affected by how the midwife listens, responds and acts. For example, in a piece about sexual abuse a woman hears the voice of her abuser echoed in the voice of the midwife providing care in labour. The exercise allows the participant to enter the psyche of the woman to achieve an empathetic response to her distress in childbirth. Compassionate care cannot be provided without this empathic engagement which should be a precursor to the kindness that women will remember and carry with them for life. In the research for this particular piece we interviewed survivors of sexual abuse, and one woman remembered her whole experience of the maternity service as 'having hands all over me'. We wanted the participants to experience this feeling and used a model to portray a woman's journey through antenatal care, labour and postnatal care sticking white cardboard hands onto the model at every physical contact point in the journey. The last hand was over her mouth showing how we can effectively silence women by not listening and by not responding appropriately to women's verbal and behavioural messages. The theatre methods we use encourage discussion and debate about complex interactions and we may not reach neat conclusions but we allow the difficult issues to rise out of the dark in order to improve every-one's experience of the maternal health services. Forum theatre, as used by Progress, allows us to practise being better communicators in order to achieve this aim.

From progress to practice with a letter of love: Gemma's reflections on Progress

Having been energized and motivated by my work using forum theatre methods as a midwife actor with Progress Theatre I looked to drive change in my local area of midwifery practice, at an acute maternity hospital in the United Kingdom. In an attempt to influence practising midwives, I developed a 45-minute workshop using theatre and storytelling that aimed to emphasize the importance of showing the same compassion to ourselves and our colleagues as we do to the women in our care.

The workshop I developed reflects my personal experience and belief that all midwives and maternity support workers are kind, compassionate and brave; even those who might have been challenging to work with were doing the best they can. My hope was to offer, through this workshop, a forum to challenge my midwifery colleagues to reflect compassionately on what may be motivating each others' behaviour, and to unpack why doing their best might not be good enough. The following outlines the features of the workshop that might be adapted in other places, for other people and differing contexts

Sharing stories

The workshop begins with a story, a reflection from practice, of a senior midwife being unkind and very unsupportive to me as a student midwife. I then ask the audience to suggest external pressures that may be influencing this midwife's behaviour. The audience are invited to stand up to visually and physically represent how those pressures would feel to the senior midwife, for example a pushing down feeling. All suggestions made become a physical representation, creating a 'network image' of the pressures midwives might face. This is a technique we use in Progress Theatre to unpick unconscious behaviours and to see each other more compassionately. I asked the audience what I could have done to make it better for the senior midwife, who was being unkind. Discussion around 'othering' and extending our tribe was facilitated, in almost every session generating solutions-based discussions around how we, as individuals, can change the culture in which we work. This worked, I believe, because I was sharing my fears and anxieties with my colleagues as their peer, from the position of a band 6 midwife who works part-time. I was willing to make myself vulnerable by revealing that, though clinical practice can be challenging and overwhelming, the aspect of my work that makes me go home and cry and not want to be a midwife is other midwives: and that's the part we can control and change. The session concludes with a love letter being given to everyone:

A love letter for midwives – written by Gemma

Dear Midwife,

'I would like a moment of your time to talk to you about your practice.' This sentence can fill you with dread. It feels like nobody talks to you about your practice unless they are criticising it or trying to change it. I want to tell you about the midwifery practice I see every time I go to work. I see brilliant, kind and clever men and women doing the best they can in ever more challenging circumstances.

The practice I would like to see is if you see one of these clever and brilliant people doing something you genuinely admire or appreciate, tell them. Tell a newly qualified midwife that her handover was really good. Tell your manager if they helped you with a difficult situation. Tell someone if you admire their suturing technique or if a woman whose care you took over praised them. Say it out loud so they know *and be specific. I bet every day one of you tells a woman in your care that they are doing brilliantly. I would extend this kindness and respect to each other and see if it makes a difference. I am a band 6 midwife who works part time and I often feel I have no power to change the systems that frustrate me but I do and so do you.*

I just want to tell you today that even on the days when you are exhausted and overwhelmed, you impress me. Even when you have a little cry in the car before you come in because you can't bear to do another 12-hour shift, I think you are magnificent. Just turning up and caring for women means you are brave and clever and kind. Being a midwife is a special and important job and you are special and important because you are doing it. You give of yourself every day to women you do not know and make them feel safe. The families of community are lucky to have you.

Thank you for taking the time to read this, I know how busy you are,

Gemma Boyd

Seeing an impact

The session was made part of mandatory training in maternity care in the local Trust, so all midwives and maternity support workers, in hospital and in the community, participated. It has also become part of the preceptorship welcome day for all newly qualified nurses, midwives, physiotherapists, dieticians and occupational therapists at my hospital. The session evaluated positively, on average rating 5/5 in written evaluations and, more importantly, kickstarting debate and small changes in practice. Many midwives fed back to me that since the session they have noticed changes to how people are speaking to each other, praising each others' work and being kinder to each other. It was my experience with Progress Theatre that gave me the confidence to put my head above the parapet and call for change, while acknowledging the magnificence of those I work with every day. Who knew one band 6 part-time midwife could make a difference in a unit that has 9,000 births a year?

Conclusion

We have used forum theatre to represent 'real-life' midwifery or healthcare scenarios, which stimulate discussion and debate around compassionate and respectful maternity care. By using actors who have experienced the situations portrayed, and by using well-researched scripts, participants report the ability to positively change practice. Being engaged in Progress Theatre, as a midwife actor, enables critical reflection and personal development by constantly working to understand how other people think and feel. We believe that theatre methods offer ideal ways for midwives to enhance compassionate care through experiencing life from other people's perspectives.

KEY MESSAGES

- Forum theatre methods can be used to explore personal experiences and organizational cultures in health services.
- Midwives and health professionals value sharing practice experiences.
- Compassionate care can be encouraged through personal reflection and shared experiences.

ACTION POINTS

- Try to find time to share positive work stories with each other.
- Give meaningful, detailed positive feedback on specific issues.
- Explore your own and others' experiences by considering motivations and external pressures/influences for challenging behaviours.

29 Moving to positive childbirth

Milli Hill

Women talking to women can sometimes be dismissed as 'gossip' or 'chit-chat', but it's at the heart of a new movement in childbirth, set up in 2012 from the living room of a passionate mum, and now boasting over 300 free-to-access antenatal groups worldwide.

In this chapter, I will explain how the Positive Birth Movement (PBM) aims to shake up birth by raising expectations, spreading awareness of human rights, and empowering women to approach birth differently. I will also describe how women in the PBM network consistently report that being treated and spoken to with kindness and respect is at the heart of a positive birth experience.

When we chat

Words are powerful; words can make a difference. Spoken or written, words can make strong imprints on us, in particular at the 'heightened' times of our life like birth and death, when our antennae are metaphorically extended to make us more receptive, and a layer of our emotional skin is missing allowing us to be more easily soothed or hurt.

Often even well-intentioned words can jar or damage at these sensitive times. 'You are only 3cm', and, 'Would you like some gas and air?' are two classic examples of words that can be given with kindness but which women often report feeling deflated by. Deeply hurtful too is the much-used term, 'failure to progress', and women are often concerned and confused by the words 'increased risk'.

These exchanges of words can be analyzed to reveal problems in the power dynamic of the birth place. Whilst they may be kindly spoken, they reveal a subtext which says, 'I understand this situation far better than you', or 'You are not performing according to our standards'. Women often come away from their birth experience with at least one of two other 'stock' phrases: 'They did not let me' and 'I had a healthy baby and that is all that matters'. They are disempowered.

It was this disempowerment that started to bug me once I had had my first baby back in 2008. Some years previously I had read and enjoyed *The Whole Woman* by Germaine Greer, in which she presents the argument that the many states of womanhood – pregnancy and childbirth being one – are pathologized, causing us to spend our entire lives, as she puts it, 'under the doctor'.

So I understood a little bit about the politics of childbirth, but as I became a mother and friends around me did too, I began to see the theory brought to life, as so many of them – myself included – planned to have a 'natural' or 'normal' birth, and ended up with quite the opposite. There seemed to be an epidemic of negativity, and amidst this, normally assertive and intelligent women were talking about their births in very disempowered terms, as if they had no control whatsoever about what happened to them, and didn't even feel they were entitled to any.

Fear of childbirth

This disempowerment seemed to be a direct result of the widespread fear of childbirth. Childbirth was a job for the 'experts', and it was unsafe for women to take anything other than a passive role in their care, so great were the risks involved. But being passive and fearful was merely leading to more negative experiences, which in turn reinforced the belief that being passive and fearful was the right approach.

I called this vicious circle the 'Fear Becomes Fact Cycle of Birth Negativity', and set up the Positive Birth Movement in October 2012 with

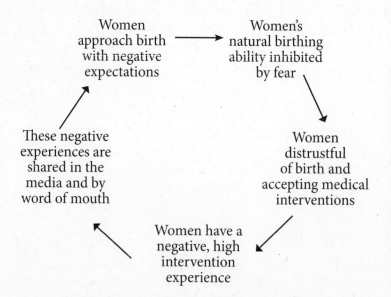

Figure: Fear Becomes Fact Cycle of Birth Negativity

the intention of breaking it. At the time I wrote:

> Often, when we try to address this loop, we focus, quite rightly, on what
> happens in the hospital... But what if we let that be, and tried to break the
> cycle at a different point? What if we challenged the information, feelings and
> negative expectations that are held in women's minds and hearts as they feel
> the first tightenings of labour? What if women walked towards the hospital
> reception with an entirely different mind-set?

Of course, in October 2012 I had no idea what a huge 'thing' I was
starting! My experience as a blogger had taught me that, when you drop
something out into cyberspace, ideas that really capture and appeal to
people have a way of taking on a life of their own, and this was certainly
a good example!

Positive childbirth

My suggestion was that women set up 'Positive Birth Groups' – free to
attend, non-judgemental discussion groups where women could gather
and share thoughts, ideas, and information relating to positive birth, all
linked together under one big umbrella by the wonders of social media.
It spread like wildfire.

Within a matter of weeks there were groups being set up all over the
UK and many more beyond. Two years later, the Positive Birth Movement
has over 200 groups in the UK, over 50 in the USA and Canada, and
many more around the world, in places as far flung as Brazil, Malaysia,
Oman, Denmark, Cyprus, Germany, Ireland, France, Holland, Turkey,
Poland, Qatar, Malta, Israel and Singapore. Our manifesto is quite simple:

> We are a grass roots movement, spreading positivity about childbirth
> via a global network of free Positive Birth groups, linked up by social
> media.

> We believe that every woman deserves a positive birth.

> *We think a positive birth means:*
> - Women are where they want to be
> - Choices are informed by reality not fear
> - Mothers are empowered and enriched
> - Memories are warm and proud

Our movement exists because, at a global level, many women are not currently having a positive birth.

We hold the birth experience to be of fundamental importance, to mothers, to fathers, to babies, to families and to society.
We wish to change birth for the better.

We aim to:
- Challenge the culture of negativity and fear that exists around birth
- Share positive birth experiences
- Share information about choices and rights in childbirth
- Encourage women to raise their expectations of childbirth

We will do this by:
- Establishing a network of free to attend positive birth groups
- Linking all groups together via social media to build a global network of shared expertise, power and positivity.
- Working together to challenge the culture of fear that surrounds birth.
- Empowering women to approach birth differently.

By simply bringing women together to talk to other women, we hope to challenge the current negative portrayal of childbirth in the media, break the 'Fear Becomes Fact' cycle, and also go some way to repair what I call the 'broken chain of wisdom' – a cultural situation in which women have not been handed down much information or positivity from their own mothers, who often gave birth in quite sterile and oppressive circumstances themselves in the 70s and 80s.

Coming together to share stories, knowledge and experience also raises awareness of women's human rights and entitlements in childbirth, an area which is so completely new that it is often barely on people's radar! *'Human rights? In childbirth?'* But it's working – as one PBM Facilitator told me recently: *'A woman wanting to have a home birth after a caesarean section (HBAC) in our area was recently told, "You're not allowed." I have been able to put her in touch with a woman who has had an HBAC in our area, through the same trust, with the same homebirth team that she is requesting.'*

This is the power of the network – in particular one that utilizes social media. Time after time women contact our Facebook page having been given a piece of advice that does not sit well with them, and within minutes they are able to access a global network of birth workers and women who have already been in similar shoes. Of course, the final course of action remains their decision, but they always report feeling empowered by the information gained, and, furthermore, deeply touched by the huge waves of compassionate support that come their way through cyberspace.

Jane Dutton @TiniestHobo · Jun 18
I will forever be grateful to the kindness of strangers over the last week. Thank you @birthpositive and @millihill and so many more.

Expand   ← Reply   ↻ Retweet   ★ Favorited   ··· More

This kind of support – just 'women talking to women' – actually has an evidence base. For example, research has shown that women with a high level of social support have better mental wellbeing during pregnancy, birth and postpartum, and a lower level of physical complications during labour and delivery.

The Positive Birth Movement itself was recently the subject of a small-scale study by academics at the University of Derby, who analyzed the responses of several women who had attended a PBM group. The study suggested that, as the baby boom stretches services, women are more in need of support and access to information, and that the PBM could play a role in this by offering women information about birth choices and sharing positive birth stories.

The study also found that 'Positive birth experiences were linked to the woman feeling as though the medics had explained her options to her and she was able to make an informed choice in relation to her birth experience. When control was taken away from the woman and procedures were performed without her consent dissatisfaction and trauma was reported.'

At the Positive Birth Movement, we hear this message every single day. It is the attitude of professionals, the words they use, and whether women feel they have made informed choices and been able to consent or not consent, that lies at the absolute heart of how women feel about their childbirth experience, regardless of the mode of delivery. Compare and contrast:

> 'As soon as I saw my midwife, I told her "I can't do this any more." She looked me dead in the eye and told me "Kate, you're doing it." That one sentence empowered me more than I can ever tell anyone.'

> 'The doctor who insisted on delivering my baby cut the cord, announced the gender and held her aloft like a hunting trophy. She illustrated her take on who was relevant in the room and who wasn't. My husband and I did not feature, let alone the baby.'

In each of these fragments in time, the practitioners involved did not think they were being kind or unkind, they were simply doing their job as they felt right and appropriate. And yet, whilst one gave all the power to the labouring woman, the other unwittingly took all of that power away.

Unfortunately, in spite of being the 'positive' birth movement we hear stories of women being disempowered and even mistreated on a daily basis, and many women who have experienced birth trauma present at our groups to debrief their stories, simply because there are currently not many other places for them to go. For this reason, we have created the All That Matters Project, where we are documenting women's accounts of everything that mattered to them in their birth experience and, in doing so, giving them a space to make their voices heard.

Many of the stories we have received so far would be an enlightening read for birth professionals, although many are harrowing. They certainly illustrate that we are a long way from breaking the 'Fear Becomes Fact' cycle, and indeed how needed a book on kindness and compassion is. In this climate, which Michel Odent has described as *'the bottom of the abyss'*, even the Positive Birth Movement itself comes under fire for suggesting that birth can be improved upon, with many women still subscribing to the view that all interventions in childbirth are necessary and that a healthy baby really is 'all that matters'.

However, those involved in our movement believe that this should be the very baseline of our expectations, and that women, babies and families deserve much better. It's clear there is much work to be done, but the fact that the Positive Birth Movement exists, and that you hold in your hand this book, shows we are making strident progress. Words are powerful; words can make a difference.

Conclusion

The Positive Birth Movement seeks to influence changes in maternity services by encouraging women to support women. What the work has taught me is that, whilst birth is an everyday event for maternity staff, for a woman in labour it is a time of huge importance and heightened sensitivity. She will remember every detail – forever. Words and actions have the ability to affect her deeply, and need to be chosen carefully. Trauma is so often worsened or even caused, not by the actual events of birth, but by the way women are treated. Professionals who have the privilege of being present when a woman has her baby need to act with huge sensitivity, and be led by their hearts.

If you are lucky enough to have this wonderful job, remember that your own personal experiences – of your own birth, the birth of your children, or births you have witnessed – shape your assumptions of what it means to give birth, how we should or shouldn't give birth, or what a woman in labour may want or need. For this reason, it's important to question and challenge your actions and attitudes regularly.

Acting with kindness, compassion and respect involves a strange mix of humility and recognition of your own huge influence. At the PBM we often hear of midwives and other birth workers who, in allowing the woman they attend to fully experience her own power in labour and birth, paradoxically become a figure of deep significance in her memory forever.

KEY MESSAGES

- The Positive Birth Movement seeks to challenge the culture of negativity and fear that currently exists around childbirth, and repair the 'broken chain of wisdom', by bringing women together to talk, share stories, and empower each other with information.
- Our network, which has a strong social media presence, as well as over 300 'real' groups in the UK and around the world, raises women's expectations of childbirth, and their awareness of their human rights and entitlements.
- Women in our network consistently report that a positive birth experience is fundamentally linked to the way they are treated and spoken to by professionals during their pregnancy and labour. Words have the ability to both empower and undermine.

ACTION POINTS

- If you are about to speak, think about the words you use. If you have any doubts that what you say may be helpful, stay silent, and listen instead. Being well intentioned does not in itself guarantee that your words or actions are kind, compassionate or respectful.
- Listen to women. Respect their views, their unique perspective on the progress of pregnancy and labour, and above all their bodily autonomy.
- Consider deeply the issues around consent. Let the woman in labour do the 'allowing'. Let her be the most powerful person in the room.
- Explain what is happening however her labour unfolds.
- Take a look at allthatmattersproject.wordpress.com. Whilst you may find it harrowing, it's important to know how your actions and words make a difference.

30 Walking in another's shoes

Gill Phillips

When delivering health services to any population, we are charged with meeting their needs, as much as we can. This chapter is about an innovative approach that aims to discover the perspective of the people providing and receiving healthcare. It is about finding ways to join things up, bringing the different parts of 'the system' together (including informal networks), to co-produce imaginative solutions that put people rather than processes in the centre. The Whose Shoes? *approach pulls no punches regarding the issues that are up for discussion; but this is welcomed in organizations genuinely trying to foster a culture of openness, collaboration and trust*

Having a baby

In the case of childbirth and maternity services, the most important and unequivocal outcome is the safety of mother and baby. But what does 'safety' mean? How do we make it a positive experience for all concerned? Does the father feel included, perhaps struggling with keen and less keen brothers and sisters? And, as a would-be Granny myself, do things start off on the right note with the wider circle of family and friends? What happens when you add to the mix all the health professionals, the policy makers, and the performance managers. So many perspectives. Such scope for over-complication – and yet we need to keep things simple; to keep them human.

Birth and death are the ultimate levellers. Every human being passes through these primeval passages into the unknown. We are at our most vulnerable and rely completely on the care, compassion and dedication of others. However, the circumstances in which we are born or die vary enormously. Some will have elaborate birth plans or end of life plans; others will blunder in or out of the world. In our search for a safe, positive experience, how can we understand what is important to different people and personalize care and support? How can we ensure that these natural, eternal events benefit from the wonderful developments in science and technology without being over-medicalized?

It seems ironic that, as our skills and knowledge increase, so does our fear of childbirth and our angst about how to measure 'patient experience'. The whole backdrop of expectations, health and safety requirements, bureaucracy, a growing culture of litigation, and shortage of money provides wonderful scope for a *Whose Shoes?* approach to tease through what really matters. And this is the project that is now in full swing (Nutshell Comms, 2014) with a Clinical Network in London supported by the Patient Experience Team at NHS England.

What are the issues?

We have an exciting opportunity to put holistic, person-centred values at the very heart of maternity practice. I believe that most health professionals come into their caring roles driven by these values but that sometimes systems, processes and pressures get in the way of embedding or maintaining these qualities in daily practice. And so we have good people – midwives and obstetricians and other professionals – working under intense pressure, a pressure to focus on risk and process women through 'the system'.

Clinical guidelines, excessive amounts of record keeping, and a feeling of being 'monitored' are amongst some of the issues constraining maternity services. No-one would deny that these are all vital to patient safety and accountability but there is always a balance to be struck. How far does the balance tip before procedures designed to protect become counter-productive, even dangerous? If highly trained professionals, often with vast experience, become overly defensive, constantly fearful of litigation, how can they apply their flair and judgement? We need to provide conditions where they can focus on what is best in this particular situation, taking into account the wishes of this particular mother.

Feeling that we are being treated with dignity and respect and offered real choice is important to all of us. It is horrible to feel totally disempowered. This seems to be the 'Number 1 message' from maternity surveys and determines how mothers and families feel about their experience of childbirth, which in turn affects the early lives of their babies. And because childbirth is such a deep and highly personal experience, negative feelings could lead to postnatal depression or cause on-going damage to the functioning and relationships of the family. So, what could be more important than to get these things right?

Much of our recent *Whose Shoes?* work has been around improving the lives of people living with dementia and helping people to 'see the person, not just the condition'. On the face of it, this is a very different area of work. The striking similarity is that we are all human beings, united by vulnerability. For most women, giving birth will be the most vulnerable time of their lives and many transferable lessons can be learnt. 'See the person, not just the condition'. Help people have a voice and express choice and control about what is important to them. Treat people with empathy, compassion, dignity and respect. Work with people rather than taking over. Never disempower someone or make them feel stupid or inadequate... Yes, these key messages from our dementia care work seem to apply to maternity services too!

The language we use

Good communication and the choice of language is key. In dementia care this often involves non-verbal communication, picking up on why people might be behaving in a particular way, often driven by fear, rather than just the words they use. Fear plays a big part in maternity care too – and it is important for medics not to play on women's fear. Mothers would do anything not to put their babies at risk, so is it fair to be told 'You are doubling the risk of your baby dying' rather than saying that refusing a particular intervention might increase the risk from say one in 1000 to two in 1000?

Central again to our work is involving 'service users' (in other words, real people!) as equal partners in shaping services, and we are including pregnant women and recent parents in our maternity project. I regularly co-present *Whose Shoes?* workshops with people living with dementia and always try to involve them as participants, as well as family carers. The informal, inclusive nature of our work and the 'leave the roles and

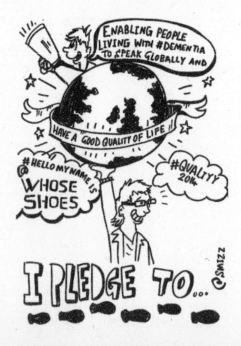

organizations at the door' approach means that a person with dementia speaks freely to people who happen to be senior policy makers or budget holders, leading to real listening and very tangible outcomes.

For example, we are currently following up a wonderful idea around peer support at the time of diagnosis put forward by Ken Howard, based on his own experience of being told he had Alzheimer's. We launched a campaign as part of NHS Change Day 2014 in the UK in March 2014 and it is attracting a lot of interest and support. We are helping forge links between people living with dementia across the world, just as this book will help to build links amongst people making a difference in global maternity circles.

Communicating for the future

Social media is a powerful way to connect people and a really important part of my work – not least my 'in my shoes' guest blog series, whereby people with many different perspectives tell us what is or isn't working well in health and social care, including innovative products or approaches. It is through social media that many of the contributors of this book have connected, building on informal networks that are such an important part of breaking down barriers and driving change in the 21st century.

Social media, used well, is like a laser beam connecting like-minded people across the world. I learn so much from social media. For example, I have learned about maternity-related initiatives such as skin-to-skin contact of mother and baby at birth, and the community-led Positive Birth Movement (Chapter 29). I can quickly pick up different perspectives on these and other key issues. To follow an issue in more depth, I take part in focused Twitter chats (#twitchats) on particular topics such as those organized by @WeNurses and @WeMidwives. If you don't already use Twitter, I hope this fires you up to seek us out and join us! I tweet (rather a lot!) as @WhoseShoes.

Conclusion

The publication of this book comes at an interesting time. The approach has so far been very well received by the maternity community in the UK. We have had some vibrant workshops as part of the pilot scheme, constantly bringing in new people and new perspectives as we build networks and generate energy through social media. There has been an emphasis on action, with people making specific pledges as to what they will do differently as a result of the sessions. There have been a lot of 'lightbulb' moments, particularly around appropriate language, as clinicians realize the effect their words can have on the women and families in their care.

We are finding that the key ingredient is devolved leadership, and we are seeking to identify the best ways to tap into the assets of local communities to deliver the transformational change required against a backdrop of increasing expectations and limited resources. We can only do this by firing people up to take ownership and to work in partnership. Exciting times indeed.

KEY MESSAGES

- We all need to work together. We need to give people time to listen, reflect and take ownership.
- Social media is a powerful way to connect people. Connecting like-minded, passionate people is a sure-fire way to empower people to build their own solutions.
- Empathy. One of the *Whose Shoes?* poems is called 'Professionals, walk in my shoes...' Try it!
- Simplicity. What could be simpler than the human longing for kindness, compassion and respect?

ACTION POINTS

- Find and connect with the right people: people who share your values.
- Light the fires of patient experience (not literally!) and seed initiatives that will grow with local ownership and sustainability.
- Work across boundaries and disciplines, looking at issues from as many perspectives as possible and really listening to others.
- Join Twitter and link up with a much wider group of people and ideas.
- Get in touch and find out more about *Whose Shoes?*

31 Compassion in the social era

Teresa Chinn

With a staggering 74% of the world's online population now using social media (Pew Research Internet Project 2014) this new social era has well and truly arrived. You need only log on to Twitter, search YouTube or search for healthcare blogs to realize that more and more healthcare professionals are becoming social media literate and starting to use social media to enhance their practice and to connect with others. But with more of us becoming attached to our smart phones, watching out for the next tweet or updating our Facebook status where does this leave compassion? The default position is that the advent of digital media cuts us off from the human race and we lose the social interactions we get from face-to-face human contact so how can a relationship with the World Wide Web foster compassion?

Sharing and showing compassion in social media

Social media is in the palm of our hand in the form of our mobile devices so it has never been easier to share our thoughts and feelings and respond to the thoughts and feelings of others. The existence of compassion within social media healthcare and midwifery communities can be best observed within open forums, eg, Twitter, blogs and YouTube as opposed to closed Facebook groups or Snapchat. This is not to say that compassion does not exist in these spaces but merely it is easier to observe in the more open forms of social media. However compassion is evident in both spontaneous and organized interactions.

In 2013 @WeNurses (a Twitter community of nurses) held an organized discussion with nurses, midwives, health visitors, paramedics, pharmacists and patients which focused on compassion and asked 'Can nurses learn compassion?' The discussion was a learning opportunity that enabled people to share their ideas and thoughts around compassion but, although it was a discussion around compassion, it didn't really show the existence of compassion within the healthcare community on Twitter. However what ensued as a result of this discussion did. In response to the #WeNurses discussion student nurse Laura Marston (2013) wrote a blog post entitled 'Compassion: too scared to care'. In this post Marston outlines how, during a placement as a student nurse, she felt she had to 'hide her compassion' and was sometimes reduced to tears. The article highlights some of the challenges we all face as healthcare professionals and, in response to this post, Twitter saw an outpouring of compassionate caring tweets supporting and sharing Marston's story. Haines (2013) then wrote a blog post in response to Marston entitled 'Compassion in care, student experience "scared to care"' which clearly articulated the compassion that exists within social media by stating 'It was so sad to read about the experience described by Laura a student nurse on a placement and her experience of feeling scared to care. The compassion she describes providing so eloquently is at the very heart of professional nursing practice, it is a skill and an art that must be nurtured, valued and recognised.'

These events clearly show the compassion that exists in social media within the healthcare community using both Twitter and blogs to share learning around compassion and also to compassionately care for one another.

Compassionate care is shown not only in these 'big' online events but also in the small quiet everyday events. When a nurse, midwife or doctor writes a Facebook status saying that they have had a bad day they need say no more, as almost immediately they are supported by their peers. If an emotional patient story is shared via a blog or YouTube video the compassionate response can be overwhelming. The sharing and showing of compassion within social media can be a big event or even the smallest thing, but there is no doubt that it does exist. Midwives and healthcare professionals are not only sharing their thoughts and feelings regarding compassion but also responding compassionately to others.

Learning about compassion

Within healthcare we are only just beginning to realize the potential of the social era for learning and continuing professional development. However, we should also consider the possibilities of social media for learning about and nurturing compassion. With the sharing of stories about compassionate care and, conversely, care that is not compassionate, healthcare practitioners can really start to understand the impact that compassion has on the people we care for and the people we work with. Dr Kate Granger's #hellomynameis campaign shows how a lack of compassion shared via a social media platform – in this case Twitter – can lead to the learning about and nurturing of compassion on a national scale. Granger (2014) states:

"I'm a doctor, but also a terminally ill cancer patient. During a hospital stay last summer I made the stark observation that many staff looking after me did not introduce themselves before delivering care. This felt very wrong so encouraged and supported by my husband we decided to start a campaign to encourage and remind healthcare staff about the importance of introductions in the delivery of care. I firmly believe it is not just about knowing someone's name, but it runs much deeper. It is about making a human connection, beginning a therapeutic relationship and building trust. In my mind it is the first rung on the ladder to providing compassionate care.'

From a few tweets about her own care Dr Granger has made a huge impact with over 13,000 people using #hellomynameis on Twitter between September 2013 and September 2014 (Symplur, 2014). Dr Granger uses a plethora of social media, including Twitter, YouTube, Facebook and blogging, to share her story on a global scale with #hellomynameis being taken up by hospitals and universities not only in the UK but also in the United States and Australia (Yorkshire Evening Post, 2014). Through the sharing of Dr Granger's story many healthcare professionals around the world are now talking about and learning how the small things, like saying 'Hello my name is…', matter to ensure the people they care for receive compassionate care.

Another huge influence in learning around compassion via social media has been the 6Cs Live! campaign. 6Cs Live! supports the delivery of the six areas of action defined by the Compassion in Practice strategy and vision based on the 6Cs – care, compassion, competence, communication, courage and commitment – which was launched by the Chief Nursing Officer of England in December 2012. Through the use of Twitter, blogs, YouTube and the 6Cs Live! hub the campaign has not only encouraged learning and sharing about compassion but also created a common language with which to talk about and share compassionate care. This can be seen most clearly when looking at tweets using #6Cs or #6CsLive (See, for example, Bennett, 2014; Foord, 2014; 6CsLive?, 2014; Queen Victoria Hospital, 2014; Caremakers, 2014; Vincent, 2014.)

There is a huge range of materials and learning being shared around compassionate care using the #6Cs and #6CsLive hashtags. However not only are learning resources and opportunities being shared but also they are being asked for (see, for example, Andrews, 2014).

Using social media to reflect on and role model compassion

Reflection can not only be a huge force for change regarding our own behaviours but also, if shared, the practitioner can become a role model and affect change within others.

Blogging is providing a forum for midwives and healthcare practitioners to reflect and share their thoughts, and compassionate care features highly. Some great examples of reflective blogs are summarized below.

Blog name	Theme of blog and how compassion is reflected
Jenny The M jennythem.wordpress.com	This blog reflects many aspects of midwifery but the author remains compassionate in her tone and language throughout her reflections.
Sheena Byrom sheenabyrom.com	The author reflects many times about compassion in mid-wifery care in this blog, not only through her own eyes but also through interviews with others.
Gas and Air gasandairblog.com	This is a very personal blog where the midwife author reflects not only on being a midwife but also on being a mother. The blog contains some birth stories which share the value of compassionate care.
6Cs Story of the Month www.6cs.england.nhs.uk	This is a collection of stories from healthcare professionals all over the UK sharing stories about compassionate care in their workplace.

Through writing these reflections the authors not only reflect on their own compassion but also serve as role models of compassion to others.

Reading reflections from the people we care for can also provide midwives and healthcare professionals with valuable insight into compassion and the delivery of compassionate care. Patient and carer blogs such as My Baglady Life by Wendy Lee which is a reflective blog written by a lady with Crohn's disease, or 38 Line Poem by Rick Bolton, a reflective blog written by a dad who has a son with cerebral palsy, can give practitioners insight into what compassion means to the people they care for.

Social media platforms like Twitter can also provide people with an opportunity to reflect on compassion as was demonstrated in a Twitter discussion on compassion organized by a Twitter community of midwives @WeMidwives (WeMidwives, 2014a). For part of this discussion see Calvert 2014, Westbury B 2014a and Westbury 2014b.)

The reflective nature of the tweets, coupled with the fact that the discussion was held in an open form of social media, meant that not only were midwives able to reflect on their own compassion but also they were able to serve as role models for the wider community. Due to the transient nature of social media we may never know the impact of such public discussions on compassion but we do know that role modelling is a valuable way to learn. Price (2009) states 'Role modelling is central to the learning experience – exemplifying practice attitudes, skills, decisions and professional reflection in ways that become accessible to the student.' By using social media to reflect on and provide a role model for compassionate care we can create learning opportunities for others.

Virtuous circles within social media

A virtuous circle is the exact opposite of a vicious cycle in that it is a process in which a good action or event produces a good result and, as the process continues, more good results happen. Byrom (2014) explores the concept of virtuous social media circles and how communities of people devoid of hierarchies (such as those developed in social media) can support one another through multidirectional open discussions. Byrom catergorizes these discussions as:

- Midwife to mother – e.g. Chelsea and Westminster Hospital's 'Ask the Expert'
- Midwife to midwife – e.g. @WeMidwives on Twitter
- Doctor to doctor – e.g. @wedocs on Twitter
- Mother to mother – e.g. Positive Birth Movement or Mumsnet

However, in reality the boundaries are not well defined, and in the open spaces that the social era affords conversation becomes transparent and open. For example, a conversation between mothers on Mumsnet about compassion shown by a midwife can be seen and read by practitioners. In addition, a conversation between midwives in the @WeMidwives Twitter community of midwives can be seen by and accessed by mothers and healthcare practitioners. The figure below shows an infographic summarizing the Twitter followers of @WeMidwives.

Although the virtuous circles on social media may at first appear to be in well defined communities, in reality they do in fact reach beyond those boundaries, as can be seen in the infographic. Therefore, when

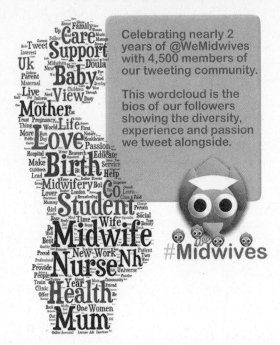

Celebrating nearly 2 years of @WeMidwives with 4,500 members of our tweeting community.

This wordcloud is the bios of our followers showing the diversity, experience and passion we tweet alongside.

#Midwives

compassion is shared in a virtuous circle on social media, not only is it shared within the community of origins' own circle but it also spreads beyond, thus sharing compassion throughout social media. Virtuous circles on social media not only support and foster compassion but also allow it to be shared across and into other virtuous circles.

Conclusion

The more we talk about, reflect on, and share compassion the more that it becomes part of our common language and ethos in healthcare. The world is changing and the social era has arrived. However, the advent of the social era does not signify a world without compassion. Compassion is being shared, shown, learnt, and reflected on in social media by midwives and healthcare professionals who also serve as role models for others. In addition, this compassion is being fostered and supported through virtuous social media circles which can reach out beyond their own boundaries into other communities.

KEY MESSAGES

- Compassion clearly exists within the World Wide Web through the human connections made via social media.

- Social media is about people, about relationships, and about connecting with people and sharing ideas, experiences and viewpoints.
- In this new social era compassion does have a place, and compassion is evident and growing within health and midwifery care social media spaces.

ACTION POINTS

- Sign up to Twitter and start or join in a conversation about compassion and reflect on your experience.
- Read one of the blogs mentioned in this chapter. How did it make you feel?
- Have a go at writing your own reflective blog about compassion. Most blogging platforms are free to sign up to. Try www.wordpress.com or www.blogger.com. Try to keep each post under 800 words in length and just explore one event or thought.
- Search for and listen in to a conversation going on in a virtuous circle. You might want to explore www.positivebirthmovement.org or search for @wemidwives or @wedocs on Twitter.

32 Kindness is a cost-effective solution

Robin Youngson

The idea that kindness could be cost-effective implies that kindness has a cost. But a midwife or doctor can perform the exact same series of tasks, in the same amount of time, whether done kindly or coldly. You don't need a staffing budget for kindness. And being kind is not an emotional burden either; those who regularly practise kindness are happier and more resilient.

So this chapter title is really shorthand for a bigger question: is management support for organizational processes that support compassion and caring a cost-effective investment? And further, should it be a priority investment in a service with budget restraints?

This question is examined from the perspective of three stories, all relating to the maternity services at Waitakere Hospital in urban West Auckland, New Zealand. The conclusions drawn from these stories are backed up with research showing the link between compassionate caring and positive outcomes for both professionals and patients, including reduced costs of care.

The context

The first story is a dramatic intervention to rebuild trust and teamwork among professionals with competing philosophies of care and fractured relationships. The focus on caring relationships led to an impressive improvement in clinical outcomes, patient satisfaction and staffing levels.

The second story is a medical error that caused severe and permanent injury to a young mother during emergency caesarean section. A courageous focus on compassion, support, honesty and open disclosure led to completely unexpected outcomes that reinforced a culture of caring and avoided expensive litigation.

The third story is a personal one: how the personal qualities of two practitioners – including kindness, respect, compassion and non-judgement – were associated with a very low rate of caesarean section and consequent cost savings.

New Zealand has a publicly funded maternity service, which is free for all citizens and permanent residents. Mothers are able to choose their own independent midwife who provides free antenatal, labour care, and postnatal care. The majority of deliveries occur in hospitals where the midwives are visiting, independent practitioners, not bound by hospital protocols. Many mothers have uncomplicated childbirth in public hospitals managed by the independent midwife, without ever seeing a doctor or other members of the hospital staff. If complications ensue, the midwife can make an urgent referral to the on-call obstetrician.

Mothers may also choose free hospital-based care provided by community midwives who are employed by the public hospital and who provide both antenatal and postnatal services in the community, and labour care in the hospital.

First story: transforming clinical outcomes through a focus on relationships

The mother had written an eight-page birth plan: no drugs, no technology, no medical interventions – childbirth was to be a mystical and rewarding experience. But progress was slow. The midwife encouraged, supported and coached the mother through a day and night of painful labour. After an hour of pushing, the exhausted mother began to despair. The midwife was concerned about fetal wellbeing and began continuous monitoring of fetal heart rate. The trace was not reassuring. Experience had taught her that calling the obstetrician would lead to immediate caesarean section. She believed that many medical interventions were unnecessary and it was her duty to 'protect' the mother from the doctors.

After another half-hour of pushing, there was a sudden and prolonged deceleration in fetal heart rate. The midwife, now fearful, called the obstetrician and reported fetal distress. It was her first communication with hospital staff. The obstetrician hurried into the room, followed closely by the anaesthetist. Grim faced, he took one look at the fetal heart rate and told the mother she needed an immediate caesarean. Suddenly there was a rush of activity. The mother burst into tears. Her husband became angry. Consent forms were thrust at the mother and she refused to sign. The midwife and obstetrician exchanged angry words. The obstetrician began to push the bed down the corridor towards the operating room while the anaesthetist attempted to complete his pre-anaesthetic evaluation. The mother, nearly hysterical with fear and pain, consented to general anaesthesia and surgery. A healthy baby was delivered. Neither mother nor father witnessed the birth of their child.

Waitakere Hospital in urban West Auckland has a busy Maternity Unit. Most of our mothers receive care from independent midwives working within the hospital's birthing facilities. Complications during labour are referred to the duty obstetrician. The unit's isolation from other acute medical services, such as intensive care, heightened professional anxiety about emergencies during labour and childbirth (since this time Waitakere Hospital has developed as a full secondary care facility). An escalating series of crises in 2001 provoked a breakdown in relationships between obstetricians and midwives. Obstetricians were extremely angry about the perceived incompetence of midwives, the 'mismanagement' of labour, and their consequent liability for adverse outcomes. Midwives, however, blamed the obstetricians for the medicalization of childbirth and the rapidly rising rate of caesarean sections.

In some aspects of obstetric care we were not alone; caesarean section rates in New Zealand, as in many other countries, have risen year on year. In 2001 the national average caesarean rate was 20.8% so when ours increased from 18% to 27%, the sense of crisis was ours. Patients suffered as professional relationships fractured in a series of 'tipping point' events: nine major patient complaints in three months; an enquiry into neonatal deaths; and an obstetrician suspended for competency review. Independent midwives refused to attend hospital policy review meetings at which clinicians questioned midwifery practice. The viability of staffing rosters was threatened as morale plummeted and staff resigned.

The conflict between doctors and midwives escalated to the national level with open hostility between the professions. Although there were apparently obvious practical solutions to our patient care problems, it was clear that resolution would only come through a process that focused on inter-professional relationships.

After a period of complete stand-off, a joint letter to hospital management from twenty-seven independent midwives gave us the opportunity to re-engage, though not before the Minister of Health became embroiled in the dispute. Midwives wrote of serious concerns about threats to their professional autonomy, women's rights, and poor relationships with obstetricians. A series of meetings exposed the high levels of anxiety, anger and blame on all sides.

We responded with a process specifically designed to rebuild trust and to focus on common goals. Known thereafter as the 'Big Day Out', we convened a one-day workshop led by an outside facilitator. Sixty-five people came, all the main contributors to obstetric care – obstetricians, anaesthetists, paediatricians, midwives, and consumer advocates. Attendance was mandatory for all the obstetricians; clinics and operating lists were cancelled and a locum obstetrician provided cover for the day.

The workshop was unusual. Carefully planned, but unscripted, it was based on role play. For most attendees this was an unfamiliar approach to learning and many were fearful. Participants role-played typical labour room crises, slowing down time to allow exploration of interactions, beliefs and difficulties in communication. Participants felt so threatened that at first roles were represented by chairs: the 'mother chair', talking to the 'midwife chair' and the 'doctor chair'.

Later in the day participants stepped forward to play their own roles, then reverse role play to explore the perspective of others. At times, the tension was electrifying. Some courageously and openly admitted their faulty assumptions and new insights. An independent midwife, acting in the role of an obstetrician, declared she had never before realized that obstetricians cared about mothers and babies as much as she did. She had believed that obstetricians were motivated just to do surgery: she now appreciated the stresses obstetricians experienced and said they deserved the support of midwives. The changed behaviour of doctors during the day was revealing but none had the courage to make such an open admission of learning.

Few promises were exchanged at that meeting. But, crucially, participants agreed to attend a monthly multidisciplinary Maternity Forum – supported by the same facilitator. Over the months Forum members continued to confront and modify beliefs about others' behaviour and received and acted on feedback about their own. The first Forum was characterized by conflict and heightened emotions. For instance, midwives vehemently defended their right to exclude doctors from the natural process of labour, while hospital specialists railed against the lack of preparation of mothers for emergency surgery and anaesthesia.

Building enough trust to identify shared goals and create an open learning environment was, in the end, helped by senior leaders openly allowing their own reactions to be explored and modified in the role of a 'vulnerable learner'. All of us had 'hot buttons' and we over-reacted to certain issues. Feedback from the facilitator allowed us to recognize our behaviour and explore the unhelpful beliefs and assumptions underlying our reactions.

After nine months (symbolically), Forum members had developed effective ways of working together and no longer required the assistance of the facilitator. Eventually this small representative group, exploring strongly held and opposing views, created collaborative solutions that made a difference. An autonomous quality improvement team was established, reporting to the Forum. An early success was resolving inter-professional conflict around induction of labour. Independent midwives agreed to allow hospital staff to manage induction, so that they could focus on supporting women in established labour. Obstetricians and midwives jointly developed the protocols for the conduct of induction. Consumers' representatives in the Forum re-wrote the patient information leaflet in simpler language. Inter-professional relationships improved and eventually an atmosphere of friendly collaboration replaced the hostility. Morale and staffing levels improved dramatically.

Patients benefited too. Although we never set explicit goals for improvement in clinical outcomes, the gains were striking. Our average caesarean rate fell by a third over the next two years, to 15.3% compared with the national rate of 22%. Our benchmarked neonatal APGAR scores equalled the best in Australasia. The percentage of five-minute APGAR scores of less than or equal to seven fell from 6% to 1%. Patient complaints fell by a factor of three.

The relative 2009/2010 cost of caesarean section versus vaginal birth in the NHS was £2,369 versus £1,665 (NICE, 2011). Our 30% reduction in caesarean sections is calculated to have saved us about £120,000 per annum in equivalent UK costs.

The total external cost of our intervention was £1,250 – the cost of hiring the facilitator. In twenty years of involvement in quality improvement and patient safety I have never seen such striking improvements in clinical outcomes, for such a tiny investment. We achieved these results because our primary focus was on the quality of caring relationships, which then allowed improvements in the clinical aspects of care.

Ten years later I left Waitakere Hospital and we had a farewell dinner in the maternity department. Among the twenty-five people at dinner were many of the doctors and midwives who participated in the 'Big Day Out'. They still deliver babies at the hospital and the warm and supportive collegial relationships persist to this day.

Second story: compassionate caring after a major patient injury

In August 2002, a terrible accident occurred in the maternity operating room at Waitakere Hospital (Waitemata District Health Board, 2002). A seventeen-year-old patient having a caesarean section under epidural anesthesia caught fire when the alcohol-based skin prep applied to her skin was accidentally ignited.

The fire burnt unseen under the surgical drapes, searing skin that was numb and anaesthetized. When the flames reached un-anaesthetized skin on the upper part of her body, the patient realized that something terrible was happening. The moment she screamed in anguish, the surgical drapes melted and everyone in the operating room became aware that a major fire was burning.

The swift action of the professionals prevented the baby from being harmed. The fire was extinguished, the patient given a general anesthetic, the surgical site was re-prepped, and the baby safely delivered. The patient suffered full-thickness, third-degree burns to 16% of her body surface. She required multiple skin grafts and is scarred for life.

I was the Clinical Leader of the hospital where this accident occurred. Over the next five weeks, I worked intensively with the General Manager and the Director of Nursing to manage the aftermath of this awful accident.

One of the stressful aspects of this experience was being interviewed on national TV news, answering the question, 'Doctor, can you explain to us how you managed to set fire to one of your patients?' I was not the patient's clinician but as Clinical Leader of the hospital I had a compelling sense of responsibility for the safety of all of our patients.

The reason I can write about this case is that all of the details are in the public domain. Back in 2002, we were one of the first public hospitals in New Zealand to employ apology and open disclosure. We believed strongly that our moral duty was to minimize further harm to the injured patient and to help her heal and recover. Honesty and openness were essential parts of our strategy.

We employed a forensic investigator and pulled together a team of enquiry comprising representatives from all the different statutory authorities. We gathered the evidence and swiftly conducted interviews with the staff involved in the accident.

We pieced together the causes of the accident. We gave daily support to the injured patient, her family, and the health professionals involved. The media scrutinized our every action – we were front-page news within a day of the accident.

In a series of media conferences, we shared our growing understanding of the causes of the accident. Before each meeting with the news media, we briefed the patient and her family and negotiated with them what could be revealed, and what kept confidential.

Five weeks after the accident, our final report was published. Both the clinicians and the hospital were exonerated. The system failures underlying the accident were widely reported and international patient safety alerts were published – many other hospitals unknowingly faced the same risk factors for an operating room fire.

The health professionals present in the operating room that day were traumatized. In many hospitals in the world, they would have been instructed to avoid all contact with the patient, deny all liability, and let the lawyers handle the fallout. In all probability the impending lawsuits would have hung over them for years.

In contrast, our clinicians had the chance to heal their wounds. They maintained a therapeutic relationship with the patient and family, making frequent visits. As the patient recovered from her injuries, so the wounds in the hearts of the clinicians healed also. Her forgiveness helped them deal with their guilt and shame.

In New Zealand, we have a national no-fault compensation scheme for injured patients; in return, patients gave up the right to sue individual health practitioners. However, patients can still sue hospitals for negligence. Even though our patient received benefits from the national compensation scheme, we believed she deserved a lump-sum payout, given the severity of her injury. We encouraged the patient to sue our own hospital, offered her legal support, and we gave her all of the reports that detailed our system failings.

The patient refused. She said that the doctors and midwives in the operating room were her 'heroes' who had saved her baby and acted courageously to prevent her from further harm in the event of a tragic accident.

Other hospitals have documented substantial financial benefits from implementing policies of apology, open disclosure and offers of compensation. The University of Michigan Health System showed a 65% reduction in lawsuits and a 59% reduction in total cost of liability (Kachalia et al, 2010).

Other than avoiding an expensive lawsuit, the cost-benefits of our compassionate leadership were incalculable. This one case profoundly changed the beliefs of medical staff; they became much more open to disclosing error and addressing patient safety risks. Apology and open disclosure became the norm. The caring culture was reflected in extraordinary levels of staff loyalty and very low staff turnover with major cost-benefits.

In the NHS, it is estimated that staff turnover and wastage costs £1.36bn per annum (The Mackinnon Partnership, 2009). Compassionate leadership and a caring culture can significantly reduce staff turnover and reduce costs. Barsade (2014a), examined the impact of an organizational 'culture of compassionate love' in long-term nursing care and showed this was associated with lower employee emotional exhaustion, less absenteeism, greater employee teamwork, higher employee satisfaction, and patients' positive mood, satisfaction, and quality of life. Even the Harvard Business Review is now publishing titles such as, 'Employees who feel love perform better' (Barsade, 2014b).

Third story: the relationship between compassionate caring and clinical outcomes

The medical staffing in the maternity unit at Waitakere Hospital is an unusual model of care: all obstetric and anaesthetic care is provided by medical specialists who work 24-hour shifts on fixed days of the week. There are no residents; specialists provide all of the medical care. The workload is sometimes onerous.

I had the privilege of partnering for many years with the same wonderful obstetrician. Every Tuesday, Raj was responsible for obstetric care and

I provided services including pain-relief in labour and anaesthesia for operative deliveries.

In 2006 I became aware that the character of the maternity unit seemed to change from day to day and this was reflected in clinical outcomes. With the assistance of a data analyst, I calculated the caesarean section rate by day of week, for a complete year of practice. The results were striking. On the days that Raj and I worked together, only 8% of labouring women had a caesarean section. On another day of the week, the average was nearly double that, 15%. An additional 5% of patients had elective caesarean section.

The hospital costs of a non-operative delivery are minimal; many patients are discharged within hours of giving birth. In contrast, most caesarean patients stayed in hospital three to five days and there are all the costs associated with surgery and post-operative care, including management of complications. The rate of caesarean section is a major driver of costs in maternity care.

On average, we did one fewer caesarean section on Tuesdays compared to the day with the highest rate, representing an annual saving of £35,000 per annum, at UK costs.

How did we achieve such a cost-effective and low rate of surgical intervention?

The first answer is that we worked collaboratively with skilled and experienced midwives to achieve safe vaginal births. Most of the credit goes to the midwives. Raj and I were both very experienced practitioners – medical specialists – but then so were all the other anaesthetists and obstetricians at the hospital. Raj had worked in Fiji and was accustomed to delivering babies without access to sophisticated hospital care. I'm sure that gave him an exceptional level of experience and confidence.

But I believe the critical factor was the compassionate relationships we brought to both patients and fellow professionals. Neither of us believed in 'difficult' patients. We did our best to practise with non-judgement, tolerance and empathy. Indeed we had more than our fair share of challenging patients. The independent midwives were very skilled in 'gaming' the system to achieve the outcomes they wanted. They saved up all their challenging and complex patients for clinics on Tuesdays, when they could rely on 'Raj' and 'Robin' to be sympathetic and flexible – and yes, relationships with midwives were on first-name terms.

Both of us brought very clear intentions to every patient: to provide compassionate and humane care with faith in the ability of our patients to achieve a good outcome. On Tuesdays, the maternity unit was calm, happy and settled.

The medical handover at 8am was telling. Some obstetricians would scan the names on the board and literally say, 'Oh I can see five caesars already!' Raj and I might see the same list of patients but our minds would be filled with all the measures we could employ to support mothers and midwives to achieve a vaginal birth with minimal complications.

All of this is anecdotal evidence. It would be wrong to suggest that the surgeon with the highest rates of intervention wasn't a caring practitioner.

But the practice of a deeply compassionate practitioner is rarely driven by anxiety. Open-hearted compassion, humility and non-judgement allow us to understand that patient outcomes are determined by many factors other than the technical skill of the doctor. When we support and validate our patients, their innate strength and healing capacity is enhanced, as demonstrated in a number of scientific trials.

The research evidence

A famous surgical study at Harvard demonstrated these effects forty years ago (Egbert *et al*, 1964). All anaesthetists were randomly assigned to conduct the pre-op surgical visit in two different ways – either in a detached clinical manner, or warmly supportive of the patient's capacity to heal, recover, and deal with post-op pain. In the post-operative period, the patients who received the supportive pre-op anaesthesia visit consumed only half the amount of morphine and they went home nearly three days earlier than patients who had the strictly 'clinical' pre-op visit.

An interesting trial in Ontario used volunteers to provide the element of compassion, in addition to 'usual' medical care. The homeless patients presenting to an emergency department who were randomized for 'compassionate contact' with a trained volunteer showed a one-third reduction in repeat emergency department visits over the next month, compared to those who had no volunteer contact (Redelmeier *et al*, 1995).

Two studies in primary care have shown a powerful association between patient-centred care and a variety of outcomes including reduced costs of care. Stewart (2000) showed that patients who received patient-centred communication subsequently recovered better, had reduced severity of symptoms and concerns, and their doctors ordered only about half the number of diagnostic tests and specialist referrals. Bertakis (2011), in a study of family physicians and general internists, showed that patient-centred care was associated with fewer visits, reduced admissions, and fewer laboratory and diagnostic tests. Patients who received the most patient-centred care had 34% lower annual healthcare costs ($948, compared with $1,435).

Other research shows the powerful impact of physician empathy on clinical outcomes and costs of care. A study of 20,000 diabetics showed that those patients who rated their primary care physicians as high in empathy had 42% fewer admissions to hospital for diabetic crisis (Del Canale *et al*, 2012).

I'm not aware of any study in maternity relating obstetrician empathy to patient outcomes but it would be a rich area to research.

Conclusion

The quality of relationships has a dramatic impact on patient outcomes but this approach to enhanced patient care is often ignored in traditional quality improvement processes. Building a supportive and compassionate organizational culture reaps handsome rewards including the potential for major cost savings. But courageous leadership is required to address issues like bullying and abuse, open disclosure, and inter-professional conflicts. Outside help may be required to facilitate processes of culture change.

Compassion and caring exist at many different levels, in the attitude of individual practitioners, in the nature of teamwork, and in the culture of whole organizations. I hope these personal stories and research findings help persuade you that investment in compassionate caring can yield major cost savings while at the same time transforming patient outcomes.

KEY MESSAGES

- There is no dollar cost for kindness or compassion.
- Investing in compassion and caring can cut your costs dramatically: you reduce staff turnover, sickness rates, and absenteeism; patient outcomes improve, complication rates fall, and overall costs of clinical care decline; an enhanced reputation will attract the best staff and improve your patient satisfaction.
- The practice of a deeply compassionate practitioner is rarely driven by anxiety. Open-hearted compassion, humility and non-judgement allow us to understand that patient outcomes are determined by many factors other than the technical skill of the doctor.
- Most managers shy away from addressing inter-professional relationships – it just feels too risky and threatening. Engendering positive relationships has the potential to improve patient outcomes.

ACTION POINTS

- Get professional help to rebuilding compassion in your department or organization. Caring and trust can be the most cost-effective investment you will ever make.

- As a leader, prepare to be vulnerable; why should you expect senior clinicians to expose their fears and vulnerabilities if you aren't willing to go there yourself.
- Make sure you reward your staff for compassion and caring, as much as you reward them for meeting production targets.

EPILOGUE:
TURNING THE SILENCE INTO A ROAR

Soo Downe and Sheena Byrom

There are only two feelings: Love and fear.
There are only two languages: Love and fear.
There are only two activities: Love and fear.
There are only two motives, two procedures, two frameworks, two results.
Love and fear.
Leunig, 2007

We chose the title of this book because we wanted to make the point that, even in countries where national policies appear to be designed to make change happen, there an untold numbers of maternity service users and workers who, every day, are experiencing distress in relation to their experiences of maternity care. To date, they have been largely silent – or silenced. We wanted this book to become a roar for these people – indeed, for all us, including you, reading our words now. We have framed it as the roar of caring and (not) cared for people trapped in a profoundly hostile space, where the inauthentic policy rhetoric of care serves only to underline the impossibility of delivering it every day, all day, day to day. We also wanted to provide real-life examples of how this situation can be changed, from people on the ground who have been there, and who have made it happen, often despite significant odds stacked against them.

The meaning of care and compassion

Soo was recently informed that in some Scandinavian countries the phrase 'maternity care' can't be translated without explanation. In English health settings, 'care' is used as a shorthand for both clinical and pharmacological provision, and for therapeutic personal and social contact. Apparently, in Scandinavian languages, these are two separate concepts; one for clinical activities, and the other for a caring attitude for delivering them. Maybe this is a metaphor: in eliding 'care' with 'techniques and services' we have lost the empathic compassionate centre of the word, which has at its root *caritas*, or love.

Kindness and caring have emotional, psychosocial, physiological and neurological effects. Indeed, recent evidence looks at the links between emotions and the neurological and immune systems, and raises the question that the consequences of these strong emotional sensations may even be epigenetic, and thus cross-generational. This, if nothing else, should inject a sense of urgency into our debate in this area.

This urgency is at the root of the contributions from our authors, and it generates a passion for change. Dictionary explanations of the origins of the word 'compassion' usually break it into two parts – 'com' (with) and 'passion'. Passion is usually traced back to the Greek 'pathos' or suffering, leading to a definition of 'compassion' as 'suffering with'. There is an intense academic debate about the differences and links between terms like 'empathy', 'sympathy' and 'compassion'. At the root of this is the claim that too much 'suffering with' leads to an inability to be objective about the nature of, and solutions to, the suffering of others.

We have not engaged with that debate in this book, as our interest in compassion is more applied. Indeed, we would like to suggest an alternative turn in the compassion discussion. If 'passion' is interpreted not as suffering, but as high and strong emotion – being passionate – then the contributions to this book become the roar of (com)passionate engagement. Addressing the toxic driver of fear that we identified in the first chapter requires being 'with passion' for change. That requires the kind of courage that is also evident in many of the contributions, and in the inspiring 6Cs from the NHS. To come full circle – the Latin origin of courage means '(from the) heart'. Back to passion again: back to roaring in the silence, so that the silence will be no more.

Where next?

This is not an academic tome. We aimed to inspire, educate and equip readers for change. If you are reading this book, you are, almost by definition, interested in this kind of change. Our line is that we need positive deviants to solve the (so-called) 'wicked' problem of a lack of compassion in maternity services. Like us, you may be fed up with the same explanations as to why we have the problem of disrespect, abuse, and lack of caring in maternity care. You may also be impatient with the default assumption that the problem can only be solved with more regulation and bureaucracy. Insightful though it was, the UK Francis report, that revealed widespread abuse in one particular NHS Trust, had 290 recommendations for change. Einstein is alleged to have said that insanity is doing the same thing over and over and expecting a different outcome. Maybe the roar behind the silence is a roar of frustration at blinkered, blanket scientific-bureaucratic approaches, which do not respond passionately to the need for us to authentically engage with those who use our health services.

If you are roaring, you are part of the solution. If only a few of you reading this take up this roar, you can make what seems to be impossible, inevitable. Indeed, it is not Them, or the System that will change this – but you, dear reader, who, with us, and with all the authors in this book, are part of Them, who are part of the System. You don't have to use up emotion and energy trying to force others to change – do it yourself, just in small things, and you will infect others positively as a result. The key points at the end of each chapter, are intended to be a pick and mix action plan, or a tool kit. Every one of us can use at least one of the tried and tested suggestions in our daily lives and practice, tailored to our specific situation.

Conclusion

As others have said before, it is easier to act your way into thinking, rather than to think your way into acting – or, more simply, *just do it!* This is not a soft and fluffy thing – it is difficult, fulfilling, challenging, and joyful. When the tipping point comes in your specific situation, as it will, the sense of achievement is overwhelming. And then the world will change.

Note from the publishers: We have made the paperback and ebook editions of *The Roar Behind the Silence* as affordable as we could in order to reach as many readers as possible. Please help us by spreading the word. You can order more copies of this book from our website (pinterandmartin.com) or contact us at info@pinterandmartin.com for bulk orders.

Contributors' biographies

Olivia Armshaw is a daughter of time, student midwife, who is discovering what it means to be a postmodern, humanistic midwife. Mother of three home-born girls. Outdoor swimmer. Brand language copywriter. Saudades do Brasil.

Sir Sabaratnam Arulkumaran is professor emeritus of obstetrics and gynaecology, St George's, University of London, president of the International Federation of Obstetrics & Gynaecology and past president of the British Medical Association and Royal College of Obstetricians and Gynaecologists.

Kirsten Baker is a senior midwifery lecturer at Oxford Brookes University. Her first degree was in English and drama and she now happily incorporates drama into her teaching as well as in the work of Progress Theatre. She is particularly interested in the emotional aspects of midwifery learning and for her MSc dissertation researched how student midwives mediate their emotional responses as they learn and adopt a professional habitus.

Alison Barrett is a Canadian-trained specialist obstetrician and gynaecologist, who currently lives and works in New Zealand. She is also a training supervisor for the Royal Australian and New Zealand College of Obstetricians and Gynaecologists.

Maria Helena Bastos is a Brazilian obstetrician/gynaecologist with a PhD in midwifery and women's health. Maria Helena is currently a national consultant for women's health at the Ministry of Health in Brazil, with strong national and international research and education partnerships to promote midwifery care.

Dean Beaumont is a father of three, and a leading expert in working with expectant and new fathers. He is the founder of the award winning programme for men, DaddyNatal, and author of *The Expectant Dad's Handbook*.

Diane Bowser is a lecturer on international health systems and economics at the Heller School for Social Policy and Management and has an appointment at the Harvard T. H. Chan School of Public Health. Her research focuses on understanding how to change incentives in order to improve health outcomes for women and children. She co-authored one of the first reports examining the evidence for disrespect and abuse experienced by women surrounding the time of childbirth.

Theresa Bourne is associate professor of midwifery and undergraduate medical studies for both Middlesex University and University College London and clinical midwife at Whittington Hospital NHS Trust. In her present role within medical school education, she is working with others on several projects to strengthen medical students' knowledge of the women's perspective and experience in maternity care, utilizing this information to strengthen kindness, compassion and respectful care.

Gemma Boyd is a midwife and clinical educator at Nottingham University Hospital Trust. Gemma joined Progress Theatre in 1999 while still a student midwife.

Anna Byrom is a senior midwifery lecturer, Progress Theatre actor and editor of *The Practising Midwife* journal. She is currently completing her doctoral studies exploring the cultural impact of the Baby Friendly Initiative on hospital cultures.

Sheena Byrom OBE is a midwife consultant and a member of the Royal College of Midwives' Better Births initiative. She lectures nationally on midwifery and childbirth related topics. Sheena was awarded an OBE in 2011 for services to midwifery, and she actively lobbies for maternity service improvements through several social media channels.

Penny Campling is a doctor, psychiatrist and psychotherapist with a particular interest in creating therapeutic environments that bring out the best in all involved. She has written extensively on healthcare culture.

Ngai Fen Cheung is a midwife and adviser to the Chinese Midwifery Expert Committee, Chinese Maternal and Child Health Association. She set up the first Midwifery Research Unit and Midwife-let Unit in China in an attempt to explain and to document the practices of midwifery both there and elsewhere.

Teresa Chinn MBE is a registered nurse and social media specialist. Teresa founded @WeNurses in 2012 as she found herself isolated from the nursing profession following years of agency nursing. The WeCommunities now connect thousands of healthcare professionals from around the world.

Michael Clift is a children's nurse working in practice development, quality, safety and research. His special interests include compassionate healthcare, clinical guideline compliance, medication errors and leadership.

Tracey Cooper is a consultant midwife. She was a member of the group for the newly updated NICE Intrapartum guideline and she is currently a midwifery advisor to the NICE Safe Staffing Advisory Committee.

Hannah Dahlen is professor of midwifery at the University of Western Sydney and a practising midwife.

Raymond G. De Vries is professor and co-director of the Center for Bioethics and Social Sciences in Medicine at the University of Michigan Medical School. He is also visiting professor at the Midwife Academy, Zuyd University and CAPHRI (School for Public Health and Primary Care), Maastricht University, Netherlands. He is author of *A Pleasing Birth: Midwifery and Maternity Care in the Netherlands* and co-editor of *Birth by Design*.

Frances Day-Stirk is president of the International Confederation of Midwives (ICM). Her 30 years of midwifery experience span clinical practice, education, maternity service management and global midwifery. She has published on a wide range of topics and presented at conferences nationally and internationally.

Soo Downe OBE is professor of midwifery studies at the University of Central Lancashire. Her research focus is the nature of, and cultures around, normal birth. Among other funded projects, she currently leads a four-year EU COST

Action (BIRTH) that addresses childbirth from a sociological, organizational, neurohormonal and epigenetic perspective. She introduced the concepts of salutogenesis and complexity into midwifery in her edited book on normal childbirth in 2004.

Ramón Escuriet is a midwife in clinical practice with two masters degrees. He is currently a PhD student, and is working with the Ministry of Health of Catalonia co-ordinating the Normal Birth Initiative project.

Julie Frohlich is a consultant midwife at Guy's and St Thomas' Hospitals, London. Julie has been a practising midwife for 30 years and has worked in several areas of midwifery including clinical (hospital and community based), education, research and publishing.

Kathryn Gutteridge is a consultant midwife who is passionate about women's issues and particularly in relation to childbearing and psychological wellbeing. She is the founder of Sanctum Midwives an organisation that educates, represents and challenges stigma around sexual abuse and its impact during motherhood.

Jenny Hall is a senior midwifery lecturer at Bournemouth University, England, who has been working in midwifery services for 30 years. Her main interests lie in educating, researching and writing about holistic and meaningful care, including spirituality, dignity and compassion.

Kicki Hansard is a recognized birth and postnatal doula with Doula UK and runs her own Doula UK approved course for aspiring doulas. Kicki is passionate about supporting and encouraging women to claim their own power by making informed choices and owning their experiences not only during birth, but in life generally.

Tamar van Haaren is a midwife and worked for several years as an independent primary care midwife as well as a hospital midwife in the Netherlands. Currently she is working as a lecturer and research midwife at the department midwifery science of Midwifery Education & Studies Maastricht, the Netherlands.

Marijke Hendrix (PhD) is a health scientist with expertise in research regarding place of birth in the Netherlands. Currently she is working as a researcher and lecturer at the Department Midwifery Science in the Faculty of Midwifery Education & Studies Maastricht, the Netherlands.

Shelagh Heneghan is a senior midwifery lecturer course leader for the post-registration midwifery programmes at University of Central Lancashire, and a Fellow of the HEA. Her interests lie in the design, implementation and evaluation of curricula that nurture the academic, practical and caring skills of students for the benefit of women and families in their care.

Milli Hill is a writer and campaigner on birth issues and the founder of the Positive Birth Movement. Her first book *Water Birth: Stories to Inspire and Inform* was recently published, and she lives in Somerset with her partner and three small children.

Billie Hunter is the Royal College of Midwives Professor of Midwifery in the School of Healthcare Sciences, Cardiff University, where she leads the Maternal, Child and Family Health and Wellbeing Research Theme. Her research focuses on exploring and enhancing emotional support and communication in maternity care.

Laura Iannuzzi is a practising midwife, recently working in one of the few Italian birth centres ('Centro Nascita Margherita') in Florence. She is an honorary lecturer in midwifery at the University of Florence and a current PhD student in health studies at the School of Health Sciences, the University of Nottingham.

Mavis Kirkham is part-time professor of midwifery at the University of the West of Scotland and holds honorary professorial positions at Sheffield Hallam University, Auckland University of Technology and the University of Technology Sydney. She has worked continuously as a midwife researcher and a clinical midwife for forty years and she is published widely.

Sue Lees is senior midwifery lecturer at Coventry University and she is also lead midwife for education and has a special interest in family planning.

Mande Limbu is the maternal health technical advisor for the Health Policy Project at White Ribbon Alliance Global Secretariat in Washington, DC. Before joining White Ribbon Alliance, Mande worked for CARE Tanzania as director of the Maternal and Reproductive Health Unit.

Amali Lokugamage is an obstetrician and gynaecologist, a medical educator at University College London Medical School and author of *The Heart in the Womb: An Exploration into the Roots of Human Love and Social Cohesion*. She works in London, UK, and is an international speaker on humanizing birth. Her lectures are published on the WHO website.

Carmel McCalmont is head of midwifery and associate director of nursing at University Hospitals Coventry and Warwickshire NHS Trust.

Sandra Morano is a professor in obstetrics and gynaecology at Genoa University and consultant obstetrician in IRCCS S. Martino – IST Istituto Scientifico Tumori University Hospital, Genoa. In 2000, Sandra created the first Italian Birth Centre, aiming to promote continuity of woman-centred care and to reduce the caesarean section rate.

Deirdre Munro is a midwife executive with the Irish Nurses and Midwives Organisation. She is also a midwife with the National Communication Project at University College Dublin.

Roberto Ortíz is a specialist paediatrics nurse and senior community midwife at the Imperial College of London Hospital.

Mercedes Perez-Botella is a midwifery lecturer at the University of Central Lancashire with an interest in women's and staff experiences of labour care. She has held different clinical and specialist posts, and published work in the area of maternity care.

Gill Phillips is the creator of the award-winning *Whose Shoes?*® concept and was named as one of the HSJ 'Top 50 Inspirational Women in healthcare, 2014' and HSJ 'Top 50 Innovators, 2014'.

Elizabeth Prochaska is a barrister and founder of Birthrights, a charity devoted to protecting women's rights in pregnancy and childbirth.

Rineke Schram is a consultant obstetrician and chief medical officer at East Lancashire Hospitals NHS Trust. Rineke qualified as a doctor in Rotterdam in 1986, and continues to work clinically as well as managerially.

Mel Scott is an occupational therapist, whose life changed when she decided it was time to become a mum. Mel shares her experiences of her miscarriage, stillbirth and pregnancy after loss to help inform professionals through her books, resources and study days at Finley's Footprints, and supports baby loss parents through her charity Towards Tomorrow Together.

Adele Stanley is a midwifery manager of the Jessop Wing's Midwifery Led Unit in Sheffield, UK. Her first degree is in Drama and English and she has always used this skill and knowledge in her teaching work at the hospital and in Progress Theatre working with midwives and health professionals.

Senga Steel is currently the deputy chief nurse at Imperial Healthcare NHS Trust in London and had held many senior nursing appointments throughout her career including assistant director of research, innovation and quality at Whittington health where this work was carried out. She also has a clinical research background and holds a PhD from University College London. She holds honorary clinical and research fellowships with both Middlesex University and Buckinghamshire New University.

Anna Ternovszky is a mother, home birth activist, and graduated as a photographer. Anna organizes parenting training with support from the government.

Kerstin Uvnäs Moberg is a medical doctor who wrote a thesis on pharmacology and a professor of physiology. Kerstin has a passionate interest in different aspects of women's health, and has researched on this topic for more than 30 years, supervised 30 PhD students, written more than 400 original articles and written four books, including *The Oxytocin Factor* and *The Hormone of Closeness*.

Lucie Warren is a midwifery lecturer and research associate at Cardiff University. Her research interests include communicating behaviour change, the psychology of lifestyle behaviours and inter-professional communication in maternity care.

Robin Youngson is an anaesthetic specialist in New Zealand, internationally renowned for his leadership in re-humanizing healthcare. He is the co-founder of HEARTSinHEALTHCARE.com, is on the editorial board of the *Journal of Compassionate Healthcare*, and is a member of the Global Compassion Council for the international Charter for Compassion.

References

Introduction: What's going on in maternity care?

Ayers, S (2013) Fear of childbirth, postnatal post-traumatic stress disorder and midwifery care. *Midwifery* 30:2 Feb pg 145-8

Ball L, Curtis P, Kirkham M (2003) *Why do midwives leave?* RCM: London. Buchan J.

Ballatt J, Campling P (2011) *Intelligent Kindness* Royal College of Psychiatrists London

Birthrights (2013) *Dignity in Childbirth: The Dignity Survey 2013: Women's and midwives' experiences of dignity in UK maternity care* London. At: www.birthrights.org.uk/wordpress/wp-content/uploads/2013/10/Birthrights-Dignity-Survey.pdf Accessed on 15.11.13

Bowser D, Hill K (2010) *Exploring Evidence for Disrespect and Abuse in Facility-Based Childbirth: Report of a Landscape Analysis.* Harvard School of Public Health and University Research USA

Childbirth Connection (2013) *Childbirth Connection: helping women and health professionals make informed maternity care decisions.* At: www.childbirthconnection.org Accessed on 11.12.13

Dahlen HG *et al* (2013) The EPIIC hypothesis: Intrapartum effects on the neonatal epigenome and consequent health outcomes. *Med Hypotheses* (2013), dx.doi.org/10.1016/j.mehy.2013.01.017

Dahlen H (2014) Managing risk, or facilitating safety? *International Journal of Childbirth* Vol 4, Iss 2

Francis R (2013). *Report of the Mid Staffordshire NHS Foundation Trust Public Inquiry* (Report) House of Commons. London. At: www.midstaffspublicinquiry.com/report Accessed on 18.10.13

Jackson M, Dahlen H, Schmeid V (2012) Birthing outside the system: perceptions of risk amongst Australian women who have freebirths and high risk homebirth *Midwifery* 28(5) 561-7

Hunter B, Warren L (2013) *Investigating Resilience in Midwifery: Final report.* Cardiff University: Cardiff.

Kirkham M (1999) The culture of midwifery in the NHS in England. *Journal of Advanced Nursing* 30, 3: 732-39.

Kirkham M (2013) Modern birth: processes and fears *Midwifery Matters* (136): 3-6

McIvor O (2013) *Turning compassion into action: a movement toward taking responsibility* FairWinds Press USA

Royal College of Midwives (2013) *State of Maternity Services Report* London. At: www.rcm.org.uk/college/policy-practice/government-policy/state-of-maternity-services/ Accessed on 17.11.13

Royal College of Obstetrics and Gynaecologists (2011) *Getting a Life: work-life balance in Obstetrics and Gynaecology* RCOG London At: www.rcog.org.uk/news/rcog-release-doctors-have-life-too Accessed on: 17.11.13

Renfrew MJ, McFadden A, Bastos MH, Campbell J, Channon AA, Cheung

NF, Delage-Silva DRA, Downe S, Powell-Kennedy H, Malata A, McCormick F, Wick L, Declercq E (2014) Midwifery and quality care: findings from a new evidence-informed framework for maternal and newborn care *The Lancet* Available at: www.thelancet.com/journals/lancet/article/PIIS0140-6736(14)60789-3/fulltext

Symon A (2000) Litigation and defensive clinical practice: quantifying the problem *Midwifery* 16 (1): 8-14

UNFPA (2014) *The State of the World's Midwifery 2014. A Universal Pathway: A Woman's Right to Health* New York: United Nations Population Fund, 2014.

Van Lerberghe W, Matthews Z, Achadi E, *et al* (2014) Country experience with strengthening of health systems and deployment of midwives in countries with high maternal mortality. *Lancet* Available at: dx.doi.org/10.1016/S0140-6736(14)60919-3 Accessed on 16.7.14

White Ribbon Alliance (2013) At: whiteribbonalliance.org/campaigns/respectful-maternity-care Accessed on 11.11.13

Youngson R (2012) *Time to Care* Rebelheart Publishers New Zealand

1 Putting relationships at the heart of maternity care

Ballatt J and Campling P (2011) *Intelligent Kindness: reforming the culture of healthcare* Royal College of Psychiatrists: London pg 33-47

Menzies LI (1959) The Functions of Social Systems as a Defence Against Anxiety: A Report on a Study of the Nursing service of a General Hospital. *Human Relations* 13:95-121 reprinted in *Containing Anxiety in Institutions Essays Vol 1* (1988) London: Free Association Books p43-88

Minkulince M Shauer PR Gillath O and Nitzberg R (2005) Attachment, Caregiving and Altruism: Boosting attachment security increases compassion and helping. *Journal of Personality and Social Psychology* 89: 817-839

Seddon J (2008) *Systems Thinking in the Public Sector*. Axminster:Triarchy Press

2 Compassion in hospital care staff

Ballatt J and Campling P (2011) *Intelligent kindness: Reforming the culture of healthcare* London, RCPsych Publications

Chambers C and Ryder E (2009) *Compassion and care in nursing*, UK, Radclliffe

Davison N and Williams K (2009) Compassion in nursing 1: defining, identifying and measuring this essential quality. *Nursing Times* 105: 36

Davison N and Williams K (2009) Compassion in nursing 2: defining, identifying and measuring this essential quality. *Nursing Times* 105: 37

Germer CK and Siegel RD (eds.)(2012) *Compassion and Wisdom in Psychotherapy* UK Guilford Press

Gilbert P (2009) *The Compassionate Mind: A new approach to life's challenges* UK, Constable

Glaser BG and Strauss AL (1967) *The Discovery of Grounded Theory: Strategies for Qualitative Research* New York, USA: Aldine De Gruyter

Kinsella EA (2007) Technical rationality in Schön's reflective practice: dichotomous or non-dualistic epistemological position *Nursing Philosophy* Volume 8, Issue 2, pages 102–113

Miles MB and Huberman AM (1994)(2nd Ed.) *Qualitative Data Analysis: An*

Expanded Sourcebook International: Sage publications

Mortimer B and McGann S (eds.)(2005) *New directions in the history of nursing: International perspectives* International, Routledge

Department of Health (2012) *Compassion in Practice Nursing, Midwifery and Care Staff Our Vision and Strategy* [Online] Available: www.england.nhs.uk/wp-content/uploads/2012/12/compassion-in-practice.pdf Accessed on 14th May 2014

NMC (2008) *The code: Standards of conduct, performance and ethics for nurses and midwives* London, UK, NMC

NMC (2014) *The history of nursing and midwifery regulation* [Online] Available: www.nmc-uk.org/About-us/The-history-of-nursing-and-midwifery-regulation Accessed on 14th May 2014

O'Brien ME (2014) *Spirituality in nursing* USA, Jones and Bartlett Learning

Seppala E (2013) The Compassionate Mind: Science shows why it's healthy and how it spreads *Observer* Vol.26, No.5 May/June [Online] Available: www.psychologicalscience.org/index.php/publications/observer/2013/may-june-13/the-compassionate-mind.html Accessed on 14th May 2014

Straughair C (2012) Exploring compassion: implications for contemporary nursing. Part 1 *British Journal of Nursing* Vol 21, No 3

Straughair C (2012) Exploring compassion: implications for contemporary nursing. Part 2 *British Journal of Nursing* Vol 21, No 4

Stationary Office, The (2013) *Report of the Mid Staffordshire NHS Foundation Trust Public Inquiry* [Online] Available: www.midstaffspublicinquiry.com/sites/default/files/report/Executive%20summary.pdf Accessed on 14th May 2014

Online resources:

- www.compassionatemind.co.uk
- www.theschwartzcenter.org

3 Dignity in maternity

Callister L (1995) Beliefs and Perceptions of Childbearing Women Choosing Different Primary Care Providers 4 *Clinical Nursing Research* 168, 175.

Chochinov HM, Hack T, McClement S, Kristjanson L and Harlos M. (2002) Dignity in the terminally ill: a developing empirical model *Soc Sci Med* Feb; 54(3):433-43.

Foster C (2011) *Human Dignity in Bioethics*. Hart Publishing, Oxford

Hodnett ED (2002) Pain and women's satisfaction with the experience of childbirth: a systematic review, *American Journal Obstet Gynecol* 186 (5 Suppl Nature) S160-72

Matthews R and Callister LC (2006) Childbearing Women's Perceptions of Nursing Care that Promotes Dignity. *Journal of Obstetric, Gynecologic and Neonatal Nursing* 33: 501

Stadylmayr W, Amsler F, Lemola S, Stein S, Alt M, Burgin D, Surbek D *et al* (2006) Memory of childbirth in the second year: the long-term effect of a negative birth experience and its modulation by the perceived intranatal relationship with caregivers, *Journal of Psychosomatic Obstetrics and Gynecology* 27(4) Pp 211-224.

Waldenstrom U, Hildingsson I, Rubertsson C, Rådestad I (2004) A negative birth experience: prevalence and risk factors in a national sample, *Birth Mar*; 31(1) Pp 17-27

White Ribbon Alliance (2011) *Charter for Respectful Maternity Care*. Available at: whiteribbonalliance.org/campaigns/respectful-maternity-care Accessed 30.11.14

4 Only for the heartstrong

Association of Radical Midwives (ARM) (2013) *New Vision for Maternity Care*. Hexham: ARM

Anonymous (2014) A call from the midwife: Why I am resigning after 10 years in the NHS. *The Independent* 08 September 2014 Accessed at: www.independent.co.uk/life-style/health-and-families/health-news/a-call-from-the-midwife-why-i-am-resigning-after-10-years-in-the-nhs-9035417.html

Ball L, Curtis P and Kirkham M (2002) *Why do midwives leave?* Royal College of Midwives, London

Beddoe A and Murphy S (2004) Does mindfulness decrease stress and foster empathy among nursing students? *J Nurs Educ.* 43(7):305-12.

Birthrights (2013) *The Dignity Survey 2013: Women's and midwives' experiences of dignity in UK maternity care*. London, UK

Davis-Floyd R (2007) Daughter of time: the postmodern midwife (part 1). *Rev Esc Enferm USP.* 41(4):705-10.

Diniz S, d'Orsi E, Domingues R, Torres J, Dias M, Schneck C, Lansky S, Teixeira, N., Rance, S and Sandall J (2014) Implementation of the presence of companions during hospital admission for childbirth: data from the Birth in Brazil national survey. *Cad. Saúde Pública*, Rio de Janeiro, 30 Sup:S1-S14

Francis, R (2013). *Report of the Mid Staffordshire NHS Foundation Trust public inquiry*. London: The Stationery Office.

Gilbert P (2009: xiii) *The Compassionate Mind* London: Constable & Robinson.

Godfrey, H (2004). *Understanding the Human Body: Biological Perspectives for Healthcare*. London: Churchill Livingstone

House of Commons (HoC) *Hansard Written Answers* for 30 June 2014

Leal M, Pereira A, Domingues R, Filha M, Dias M, Nakamura-Pereira M, Bastos M and Gama S (2014) Obstetric interventions during labor and childbirth in Brazilian low-risk women. *Cad. Saúde Pública* [online] 2014, vol.30, suppl.1

Leal M (2012) Birth in Brazil: national survey into labour and birth. *Reproductive Health* 2012, 9:15

Kitzinger S (2012) *Birth and Sex: The power and the passion*. London: Pinter & Martin.

Kloosterman, G (1982) Universal Aspects of Birth: Human Birth as a Socio-psychosomatic Paradigm. *Journal of Psychosomatic Obstetrics and Gynecology* 1, no. 1 (1982): 35-41.

Ministry of Justice (MoJ) (2013) *An Overview of Sexual Offending in England and Wales Statistics bulletin* Accessed August 2014 at: www.gov.uk/government/uploads/system/uploads/attachment_data/file/214970/sexual-offend-ing-overview-jan-2013.pdf

Multi professional education and training budget monitoring returns (2014) www.publications.parliament.uk/pa/cm201415/cmhansrd/cm140630/text/140630w0006.htm#14070173000026)

Neff K (2011) *Self Compassion*. London: Hodder & Stoughton

Sandall J, Soltani H, Gates S, Shennan A and Devane D (2013) Midwife-led continuity models versus other models of care for childbearing women. *Cochrane Database of Systematic Reviews* 2013, Issue 8.

Shapiro S, *et al* (2005). Mindfulness-Based Stress Reduction for Health Care Professionals: Results from a Randomized Trial. *International Journal of Stress Management* 12(2), p164-176.

White Ribbon Alliance (2011) *Respectful maternity Care: The universal rights of childbearing women.* Accessed at whiteribbonalliance.org.s112547.gridserver.com/wp-content/uploads/2013/05/Final_RMC_Charter.pdf

7 Don't forget Dad!

Cohen R, Lange L and Slusser W (2012) A description of a male-focused breast-feeding promotion corporate lactation program, *Journal of Human Lactation*, 18(1), 61–65

Department of Health (2011) *Views on the Maternity Journey and Early Parenthood.* London

NICE (2008) *Antenatal care: routine care for the healthy pregnant woman.* London

Wolfberg AJ, Michels KB, Shields W, O'Campo P, Bronner Y and Bienstock J (2014) Dads as breastfeeding advocates: results from a randomised controlled trial of an educational intervention *American Journal of Obstetrics and Gynaecology*, 191(3), (2004), 708–712

8 Through the eyes of a doula

Klaus MH, Kennell JH and Klaus PH (1993) *Mothering the Mother: How a Doula Can Help You Have a Shorter, Easier and Healthier Birth.* Perseus Books, Massachusetts

9 Promoting normal birth: courage through compassion

Cooper T and Lavender T (2013) Women's Perceptions of a Midwife's Role: An Initial Investigation. *British Journal of Midwifery* Vol. 21, Iss. 4, 04 Apr 2013, pp 264 - 273

Ekman P (2003) *Emotions Revealed: Recognising Faces and Feelings to improve communication and emotional life.* New York, NY: Henry Holt & Company.

Goetz J, Dacher K and Emiliana S (2010) Compassion: An Evolutionary Analysis and Empirical Review *Psychological Bulletin* 136 (3): 351–374. doi:10.1037/a0018807

Hoffman M (1981) Is altruism part of human nature? *Journal of Personality and Social Psychology* 40 (1): 121–137. doi:10.1037/0022-3514.40.1.121

Hatfield E, Cacioppo J (1993) Emotional Contagion *Current Directions in Psychological Sciences* 2: 96–99. doi:10.1111/1467-8721.ep10770953

NICE (2014) Intrapartum Care: Care of Healthy Women and Babies During Childbirth. *Clincal guideline* 190. December 2014. www.nice.org.uk

11 We can learn to be caring

Fredrickson B (2010) *Positivity: groundbreaking research to release your inner optimist and thrive*. Richmond: Oneworld

Egbert LD, Battit GE, Welch CE, Bartlett MK. (1964) Reduction of Postoperative Pain by Encouragement and Instruction of Patients. A Study of Doctor-Patient Rapport. *The New England Journal of Medicine*. 1964;270:825-7.

Youngson R. *Time to Care: How to love your patients and your job*. (2012) Raglan: Rebelheart Publishers

12 Human rights principles in maternal health

Birthrights (2013) *Response to the Care Quality Commission consultation on changes to the ways the CQC regulates, inspects and monitors care services.* Available from Birthrights: www.birthrights.org.uk Accessed 30.11.14

Bowser D, Hill K. (2010) *Exploring Evidence for Disrespect and Abuse in Facility-Based Childbirth: Report of a Landscape Analysis*. Harvard School of Public Health and University Research. Available from: www.mhtf.org/wp.../Respectful_Care_at_Birth_9-20-101_Final.pdf Accessed 30.11.14

Center for Reproductive Rights (CRR), Federation of Women Lawyers--Kenya (FIDA) (2007) *Failure to Deliver: Violations of Women's Human Rights in Kenyan Health Facilities*. Available from: reproductiverights.org/en/document/failure-to-deliver-violations-of-womens-human-rights-in-kenyan-health-facilities

Center for Reproductive Rights (CRR) (2008) *Broken Promises: Human Rights, Accountability and Maternal Death in Nigeria*. Available from: www.tractionproject.org/...skilled.../broken-promises-human-rights- accountability-and-maternal-death-nigeria

Declaration of the Elimination of Violence Against Women (1993) Article 1. Available from: www.un.org/documents/ga/res/48/a48r104.htm

d'Oliveira AF, Pires Lucas, Diniz SG, Schraiber LB (2002) Violence against women in health-care institutions: an emerging problem. *Lancet* 359(9318):1681-1685.

Economic and Social Council (2014) *Millennium Development Goals and post-2015 Development Agenda* Available at: www.un.org/en/ecosoc/about/mdg.shtml Accessed 30.11.14

Family Care International (2003) *Care-Seeking During Pregnancy, Delivery, and the Postpartum Period: A Study in Homabay and Migori Districts*, Kenya Available from www.tractionproject.org/resources/access-skilled-care/care-seeking-during-pregnancy-delivery-and-postpartum-period-study Accessed 30.11.14

Freedman L, Kruk M (2014) Disrespect and abuse of women in childbirth: challenging the global quality and accountability agendas. *Lancet* 384, 9948, e42 - e44

Gostin L, Hodge JG, Valentine N, Nygren-Krug H 2003. *The Domains of Health Responsiveness – A Human Rights Analysis* Available from: www.who.int/hhr/Series_2%20Responsiveness.pdf Accessed 30.11.14

Human Rights Watch Burundi (2006) *A High Price to Pay. Detention of Poor Patients in Hospitals.* 18, No. 8A Available from: www.hrw.org/reports/2006/burundi0906/ Accessed 30.11.14

International Covenant on Civil and Political Rights (ICCPR) (1966) Article 7 Available from: treaties.un.org/doc/Publication/UNTS/Volume%20999/volume-999-I-14668-English.pdf

Jewkes R, Abrahams N, Mvo Z (1998) Why do nurses abuse patients? Reflections from South African obstetric services *Social Science & Medicine* 47(11):1781-1795

Kayongo M, Esquiche E, Luna MR, Frias G, Vega-Centeno L, Bailey P (2006) Strengthening emergency obstetric care in Ayacucho, Peru. *International Journal of Gynecology & Obstetrics* 92(3):299-307

Kruk ME, Paczkowski M, Mbaruku G, Pinho HD, Galea S (2009) Women's Preferences for Place of Delivery in Rural Tanzania: A Population-Based Discrete Choice Experiment. *American Journal of Public Health* 99:1666-1672.

The Population Council (2014) *Confronting Disrespect and Abuse during Childbirth in Kenya. The Heshima Project.* Available from: www.popcouncil.org/uploads/pdfs/2014RH_HeshimaBrief.pdf Accessed on 30.11.14

The U.S. Agency for International Development (2014) *Maternal Health Vision for Action* Available at: www.usaid.gov/what-we-do/global-health/maternal-and-child-health/maternal-health-vision-action Accessed on 30.11.14

World Health Organization (2012) *Trends in Maternal Mortality: 1990–2010. WHO, UNICEF, UNFPA and the World Bank estimates* Available from: www.who.int/reproductivehealth/publications/monitoring/9789241503631/en/ Accessed 30.11.14

WHO, UNICEF (2014) Every *Newborn: an action plan to end preventable deaths: Executive summary.* Geneva: World Health Organization

13 What does oxytocin have to do with kindness?

Burbach JPH, Young LJ, & Russell JA (2006). Oxytocin: Synthesis, Secretion and Reproductive Functions Knobil and Neill´s Physiology of Reproduction (3 ed.): Elsevier.

Campbell D, Scott KD, Klaus MH, & Falk M (2007). Female relatives or friends trained as labor doulas: outcomes at 6 to 8 weeks postpartum. *Birth*, 34(3), 220-227.

Eriksson M, Lindh B, Uvnas Moberg K, & Hokfelt T (1996). Distribution and origin of peptide-containing nerve fibres in the rat and human mammary gland. *Neuroscience*, 70(1), 227-245.

Uvnäs Moberg K (2012). *The Hormone of Closeness* London: Pinter & Martin Ltd.

Uvnås Moberg K, Prime D (2013). Oxytocin effects in mothers and infants during breastfeeding. *Infant* 9(6), 201-206.

Puder BA, Papka RA (2001). Hypothalamic paraventricular axons projecting to the female rat lumbosacral spinal cord contain oxytocin immunoreactivity. *J. Neurosci Res.* 64 (1), 53-63.

Sato Y, Hotta H, Nakayama H, Suzuki H (1996). Sympathetic and parasympathetic regulation of the uterine blood flow and contraction in the rat. *J. Auton Nerv Syst* 59 (3) 151-158.

14 Spirituality and compassion in maternity care

Ballatt J and Campling P (2011) *Intelligent kindness: reforming the culture of healthcare* London, RCPsych Publications

Crawford P, Brown B Kvangarsnes M and Gilbert P (2014) The design of compassionate care *Journal of Clinical Nursing* doi: 10.1111/jocn.12632

Frankl VE (1984) *Man's Search for Meaning.* New York: Simon and Schuster;

Hall J (2011) *What is spiritual care in relation to women, babies and families?* Paper presented at 5th international student conference on Spiritual Care and health Professions: Context and Practice European Spirituality Research Network for Nursing and Midwifery, Amsterdam.

Hall J (2012) *The essence of the art of a midwife: holistic, multidimensional meanings and experiences explored through creative inquiry* Unpublished EdD thesis, University of The West of England Available from: eprints.uwe.ac.uk/16560 Accessed 24/05/2014

Hall J (2013) Spiritual care: enhancing meaning in pregnancy and birth *The Practising Midwife* 16(11):26-7.

Klassen PE (2001) *Blessed events: religion and home birth in America.* Princeton, NJ, Princeton University Press

Lundmark M (2007) Vocation in Theology-Based Nursing Theories. *Nursing Ethics* 14 (6), pp.767-780

Mollart L, Skinner VM, Newing C, and Foureur M (2011) *Factors that may influence midwives work-related stress and burnout Women and Birth* [online] Available from: download.journals.elsevierhealth.com/pdfs/journals/1871-5192/PIIS1871519211002058.pdf [accessed 12/12/12]

NHS Education for Scotland (2010) *Spiritual care matters: an introductory resources for all NHS Scotland staff* Available from: www.nes.scot.nhs.uk/education-and-training/by-discipline/spiritual-care/about-spiritual-care/publications/spiritual-care-matters-an-introductory-resource-for-all-nhs-scotland-staff.aspx Accessed 25/05/2014

Watson J (2008) *Nursing: the Philosophy and Science of Caring.* Denver: University Press of Colorado

Yoder EA (2010) Compassion fatigue in nurses *Applied Nursing Research* 23(4) 191-197

15 Stop the fear and embrace birth

Beck CT, Gable RK, Sakala C, & Declercq ER (2011) Posttraumatic Stress Disorder in New Mothers: Results from a Two-Stage U.S. National Survey. *Birth*, 38(3), 216-227.

Birthplace in England Collaborative Group (2011) Perinatal and maternal outcomes by planned place of birth for healthy women with low risk pregnancies: the Birthplace in England national prosective cohort study. *BMJ*, 343 doi: 10.1136/bmj.d7400.

Copeland F, Dahlen HG, & Homer CE (2013) Conflicting Contexts: Midwives interpretation fo childbirth through photo elicitation. *Women and Birth*, Available online 25th December 2013.

Curtis P, Ball L, & Kirkham M (2006) Why do midwives leave? (Not) being the kind of midwife you want to be. *British Journal of Midwifery*, 14(1), 27-31.

Dahlen H (2010) Undone by fear? Deluded by trust? *Midwifery*, 26(2), 156-162.

Dahlen H (2012) *Dancing in the grey zone between normality and risk* (conference paper). Paper presented at the Normal Labour and Birth: 7th International Research Conference

Dahlen H, Tracy S, Tracy MB, Bisits A, Brown C, & Thornton C. (2014) Rates of obstetric intervention and associated perinatal mortality and morbidity among low-risk women giving birth in private and public hospitals in NSW (2000–2008): a linked data population-based cohort study. *BMJ Open*, 2014;4:e004551. doi:10.1136/bmjopen-2013-004551.

Dahlen HG (2014) Managing Risk or Facilitating Safety? *International Journal of Childbirth*, 4(2), 66-68.

Dahlen HG, & Caplice S (2014) What do midwives fear? *Women and Birth*, Online dx.doi.org/10.1016/j.wombi.2014.06.008.

Dahlen HG, Tracy S, Tracy M, Bisits A, Brown C & Thornton C (2012) Rates of obstetric intervention among low-risk women giving birth in private and public hospitals in NSW: a population-based descriptive study. *BMJ Open*, 2:e001723 doi:10.1136/bmjopen-2012-001723.

Davis-Floyd R, & Cheyney M (2009) Birth and the big bad wolf: an evolutionary perspective. In Selin H & Srtone P (Eds.), In *Childbirth across cultures: Ideas and practices in pregnancy, childbirth and the postpartum*: Springer.

Department of Health UK (2014) *Women to benefit from £10 million for better maternity environments* www.gov.uk/government/news/women-to-bene-fit-from-10-million-for-better-maternity-environments.

Dijkstra K, Pieterse M, & Pruyn A (2006) Physical environmental stimuli that turn healthcare facilities into healing environments through psychologically mediated effects: systematic review. *Journal of Advanced Nursing*, 56(2), 166-181.

Fisher SC, Kim SY, Sharma AJ, Rochat R, & Morrow B (2013) Is obesity still increasing among pregnant women? Prepregnancy obesity trends in 20 states, 2003–2009. *Preventative Medicine* 56(6), 372-378.

Foucault M (1977) *Discipline and punish*. London: Penguin.

Gibbons L, Belizán JM, Lauer JA, Betrán AP, Merialdi M, & Althabe F. (2010). *The Global Numbers and Costs of Additionally Needed and Unnecessary Caesarean Sections Performed per Year: Overuse as a Barrier to Universal Coverage*. Geneva: World Health Organisation.

Gutteridge K (2013) Assessing progress through labour using midwifery wisdom. *Essentially MIDIRS*, 4(3), 17-22.

Gutteridge K (2014) *Clinical Outcomes Report over 3 Years - Serenity & Halcyon Birth Centres*. Sandwell & West Birmingham Hospitals NHS Trust.

Hammond A, Foureur M, Homer CS, & Davis D (2013) Space, place and the midwife: Exploring the relationship between the birth environment, neurobiology and midwifery practice. *Women and Birth*, 26, 277-281.

Hodnett ED, Downe S, & Walsh D (2012) Alternative versus conventional institutional settings for birth. *Cochrane Database of Systematic Reviews*, Issue 8. Art. No.: CD000012. DOI: 10.1002/14651858.CD000012.pub4.

Hodnett ED, Gates S, Hofmeyr GJ, & Sakala C (2013) Continuous support for women during childbirth. *Cochrane Database of Systematic Reviews*, Issue 7. Art. No.: CD003766. DOI: 10.1002/14651858.CD003766.pub5.

Jackson M, Dahlen H, & Schmied V (2012) Birthing outside the system: Perspectives of risk amongst Australian women who have high risk homebirths. *Midwifery*, 28(5), 561-567.

Jordan K, Fenwick J, Slavin V, Sidebotham M, & Gamble J (2013). Level of burnout in a small population of Australian midwives. *Women and Birth*, 26(2), 125-132.

LeDoux JE, Romanski L, & Xagoraris A (1989). Indelibility of subcortical memories. *Journal of Cognitive Neuroscience*, 1, 238-243.

Li Z, Zeki R, Hilder L, & Sullivan EA (2012). Australia's mothers and babies 2010. *Perinatal statistics series* no. 27. Cat. no. PER 57.

Main E, & Menard K (2013). Maternal mortality: Time for national action. *Obstetrics and Gynecology* 122(4), 735-736.

Maslach C, Schaufeli WB, & Leiter MP (2001). Job burnout. *Annual Review of Psychology*, 52(397), 422.

Merrick S (2013) Who's Afraid of the Big Bad Birth *AIMS Journal*, 25(3), 20.

Mills TA, & Lavender T (2011) Advanced Maternal Age. Obstetrincs, *Gynaecology & Reproductive Medicine*, 21(4), 107-111.

Morris T, & McInerney K.(2010) Media Representations of Pregnancy and Childbirth: An Analysis of Reality Television Programs in the United States. *Birth*, 37(2), 134-140.

Murphy-Lawless J (1998) *Reading Birth and Death: A History of Obstetric Thinking*. Bloomington and Indianapolis: Indiana University Press.

Nieminen K, Stephansson O, & Ryding EL (2009) Women's fear of childbirth and preference for cesarean section – a cross-sectional study at various stages of pregnancy in Sweden. *Acta Obstetrica et Gynecology* 88(7), 807-813.

Odent M (1999). *The Scientification of Love*. London: Free Association Books.

Otely H (2011). Fear of childbirth: understanding the causes, impact and treatment. *British Journal of Midwifery*, 19(4), 215-220.

Powell Kennedy H, & Shannon, MT (2004). Keeping birth normal: Research findings on midwifery care during childbirth. *JOGNN - Journal of Obstetric, Gynecologic, & Neonatal Nursing*, 33(5), 554-560.

Priddis H, Dahlen H, & Schmied V (2012). What are the facilitators, inhibitors, and implications of birth positioning? A review of the literature. *Women and Birth*, 25(2), 100-106.

Priddis H, Dahlen H, & Schmied V (2011). Juggling Instinct and Fear: An Ethnographic Study of Facilitators and Inhibitors of Physiological Birth Positioning in Two Different Birth Settings. *International Journal of Childbirth*, 1(4), 227-241.

Quirk GJ, Repa JC, & LeDoux JE (1995). Fear conditioning enhances short-latency auditory responses of lateral amygdala neurons: Parallel recordings in the freely behaving rat. *Neuron*, 15, 1029-1039.

Regan M, & Liaschenko J (2007). In the mind of the beholder: Hypothesized effect of intrapartum nurse's cognitive frames of childbirth caesarean section rates. *Qualitative Health Research*, 17(5), 612-634.

Rouhe H, Salmela-Aro K, Toivanen R, Tokola M, Halmesmaki E, & Sisto T (2012). Obstetric outcome after intervention for severe fear of childbirth in nulliparous women – randomised trial. *BJOG*, 120(1), 75-84.

Sandall J, Soltani H, Gates SAS, & Devane D (2013). Midwife-led continuity models versus othermodels of care for childbearing women. *Cochrane Database of Systematic Reviews*, Issue 8. Art. No.: CD004667. DOI: 10.1002/14651858.CD004667.pub3.

Schindler Rising S, Powell Kennedy H, & Klima C (2004). Redesigning prenatal care through CenteringPregnancy. *Journal of Midwifery and Women's Health*, 49(5), 398-404.

Schott J, Henley A, & Kohner N (2007). *Pregnancy, loss and the death of a baby: guidelines for professionals* (3rd ed.). Shepperton on Thames: Bosun Press.

Schryer LeBel F (2008). *Stress and Burnout in Canadian Midwives*. Saint Mary's University, Halifax

Selanders LC (2010). The power of environmental adaptation: Florence Nightingale's original theory for nursing practice. *J Holist Nurs*, 28(1), 81-88.

Simkin, P (1992). Just another day in a woman's life? Part II: Nature and consistency of women's long-term memories of their first birth experiences. *Birth*, 19(2), 64-81.

Sutton J (2000). Occipito-posterior positioning and some ideas about how to change it. *The Practising Midwife*, 3(6), 20-22.

Teate A, Dahlen H, Virginia S, Lamb K, Swain J, Garland D, *et al* (2013). Reporting on the observational data in the midwives and women's Interaction study (MAWI) - Exploring their interactions during antenatal consultations. *Women and Birth*, 26: S22-S42. dx.doi.org/10.1016/j.wombi.2013.08.213.

Uvnäs Moberg K (2003) *The Oxytocin Factor*. London: Pinter & Martin.

Wagner M (2001). Fish can't see water: the need to humanize birth. *International Journal of Gynaecology and Obstetrics*, 75(Suppl 1), S25-37.

Walsh D & Gutteridge K (2011) Using the birth environment to maximise women's potential in labour. *MIDIRS Midwifery Digest* 21(2).

Woods M (1982). *Aristotle's Eudemian Ethics*. Cambridge: Clarendon Press.

16 How environment and context can influence capacity for kindness

Ball L, Curtis P and Kirkham M (2002) *Why Do Midwives Leave?* Royal College of Midwives, London.

Bolton G (1999) *The therapeutic potential of creative writing. Writing myself.* London, Jessica Kingsley

Bolton G (2001) *Reflective practice. Writing and professional development*. London, Paul Chapman

Brodie P and Homer C (2009) 'Transforming the culture of a maternity service; St Georges Hospital, Sydney Australia.' Davis-Floyd R, Barclay L, Davies BA and Tritten J *Birth Models that Work*. Berkeley, University of California Press.

Deery R (2008) The tyranny of time: tensions between relational time and clock time in community-based midwifery. *Social Theory and Health* 6, 4; 342-363.

Department of Health (1993) *Changing Childbirth: Report of the Expert Maternity Group*. London, HMSO.

Dixon NM (1998) *Dialogue at Work; making talk developmental for people and organisations*. London, Lemos and Crane.

Garratt EF (2010) *Survivors of Childhood Sexual Abuse and Midwifery Practice* Oxford, Radcliffe.

Homer C, Brodie P and Leap N (2001) *Establishing Models of Continuity of Midwifery Care in Australia. A Resource for Midwives*. Sydney, University of Technology Sydney, Centre for Family Health and Midwifery.

Homer C, Brodie P and Leap N (2008) *Midwifery Continuity of Care: A Practical Guide*. Sydney, Churchill Livingstone, Elsevier.

Johns C (2004) *Being Mindful*, Easing Suffering London, Jessica Kingsley

Kenworthy D and Kirkham M (2011) *Midwives Coping with Loss and Grief: stillbirth, professional and personal losses* London, Radcliffe

Kirkham M (1999) The culture of midwifery in the NHS in England. *Journal of Advanced Nursing* 30, 3: 732-39.

Kirkham M (2010) In fear of difference, in fear of excellence. *The Practicing Midwife* 13,1; 13-15.

Kirkham M, Morgan RM and Davies C (2006) *Why Midwives Stay* London, Department of Health and University of Sheffield.

Kirkham M, Stapleton H, Curtis P and Thomas G (2002) Stereotyping as a professional defence mechanism. *British Journal of Midwifery* 10, 9: 509-513

Lipsky M (1980) *Street-Level Bureaucracy: Dilemmas of the Individual in Public Services*. New York, Russell Sage Foundation.

Macy J and Johnstone C(2012) *Active Hope: How to face the mess we're in without going crazy*. New World Publishers

Menzies Lyth I (1988) *Containing Anxiety in Institutions. Selected Essays Vol 1*. London, Free Association Books.

Midwives (2014) news item Caseload Caring Midwives 2014,3;54

NICE (2014) *Intrapartum guidelines*. Available from: www.nice.org.uk/guidance/CG190. Accessed December 3rd 2014

Rosenberg MB (2003) *Nonviolent Communication: a language for life*. Encinitas, California, Puddle Dancer Press.

Williams R (2014) What the Body Knows *Resurgence and Ecologist* 2014 March/April: 34-35.

Youngson R (2012) *Time to Care*. Raglan, New Zealand, Rebelheart

17 Caring for ourselves

Hart A, Blincow D, & Thomas, H (2007) *Resilient therapy: Working with children and families*. Hove: Routledge.

Hodges HF, Keeley AC, & Troyan PJ (2008) Professional resilience in baccalaureate-prepared acute care nurses. *Nursing Education Research*, 29(2), 80-89.

Hunter B (2006) The importance of reciprocity in relationships between community-based midwives and mothers. *Midwifery*, 22(4), 308-322.

Hunter B, & Warren L (2013). *Investigating resilience in midwifery: Final report*. Cardiff: Cardiff University.

Hunter B, & Warren L (2014) Midwives experience of workplace resilience. *Midwifery*, 30(5). 926-934.

Jacelon CS (1997) The trait and process of resilience. *Journal of Advanced Nursing*, 25(1), 123-129.

Jackson D, Hutchinson M, Everett B, Mannix J, Weaver R, & Salamonson Y. (2011) Struggling for legitimacy: Nursing students' stories of organisational aggression, resilience and resistance. *Nursing Inquiry*, 18(2), 102-110.

McAllister M, & Mckinnon J (2009) The importance of teaching and learning resilience in the health disciplines: A critical review of the literature. *Nurse Education Today*, 29(4), 371-379.

McCann CM, Beddoe E, McCormick K, Huggard P, Kedge S, Adamson C, & Huggard J (2013) Resilience in the health professions: A review of recent literature. *International Journal of Wellbeing*, 3(1), 60-81.

Ungar, M (2012) Social ecologies and their contribution to resilience In M. Ungar (Ed.), *The social ecology of resilience: A handbook of theory and practice*. New York: Springer

18 Clinical guidelines

Birthrights (2013) *Human rights in maternity care*. Available at: www.birthrights.org.uk/ Accessed 20 June 2013

Birthrights (2013) *The end of independent midwifery? Consultation launched into mandatory insurance for midwives*. Available at: www.birthrights.org.uk/2013/02/the-end-of-independent-midwifery-consultation-launched-into-mandatory-insurance-for-midwives/ Accessed 30 May 2013

Department of Health (DH) (2012) *Liberating the NHS: no decision about me, without me*. Government response. London; DH.

Department of Health (DH) (2013) *Patients first and foremost. The initial government response to the Report of The Mid Staffordshire NHS Foundation Trust Public Inquiry*. London: DH.

General Medical Council (2008) *Consent: patients and doctors making decisions together* Available at: www.gmc-uk.org/guidance/ethical_guidance/consent_guidance_index.asp (accessed 18.07.2014)

General Medical Council (2013) *Good Medical Practice – The duties of a doctor registered with the General Medical Council* www.gmc-uk.org/guidance/good_medical_practice/duties_of_a_doctor.asp Accessed 18.07.2014

Greenhalgh T, Howick J, Maskrey N (2014) Evidence based medicine: a movement in crisis? *BMJ*. 2014; 348: g3725. Available at: www.ncbi.nlm.nih.gov/pmc/articles/PMC4056639/ Accessed on 30.11.14

Haslam D (2014) www.england.nhs.uk/revalidation/ro/train-net/

Hurwitz B (1999) Legal and political considerations of clinical practice guidelines *BMJ* 1999;318:661–4

Hurwitz B (2004) How does evidence based guidance influence determinations of medical negligence? *BMJ* 2004;329:1024

Joyce R (2012) *The unlikely pilgrimage of Harold Fry*. London: Doubleday: 181.

Kitzinger S (2006) *Birth crisis*. Abingdon: Routledge.

National Collaborating Centre for Women's and Children's Health (NCCWCH) (2007) *Intrapartum care: care of healthy women and their babies during childbirth*. London: RCOG Press.

Nursing and Midwifery Council (NMC) (2006) *Standards for the preparation and practice of supervisors of midwives*. London: NMC

Nursing and Midwifery Council (NMC) (2008) *The code: standards of conduct, performance and ethics for nurses and midwives*. London: NMC

Nursing and Midwifery Council (NMC) (2012) *Midwives rules and standards 2012*. London: NMC.

Royal College of Obstetricians and Gynaecologists (RCOG) (2010) *Understanding how risk is discussed in healthcare: information for you*. London: RCOG Press.

Sackett DL, Rosenberg WMC, Gray JAM *et al* (1996) Evidence based medicine: what it is and what it isn't. *BMJ* 312(7023):71.

19 Making it happen in China

Cheung NF, Mander R, Wang X, Fu W, Zhou H, Zhang L (2011a) Clinical outcomes of the first midwife-led normal birth unit in China: a retrospective cohort study *Midwifery* 27:582-587, DOI:10.1016/j.midw.2010.05.012 dx.doi.org/10.1016/j.midw.2010.05.012 accessed 18.1.2011

Cheung NF, Mander R, Wang X, Fu W, Zhou H, Zhang L (2011b) Views of Chinese women and health professionals about the midwife-led care in China. *Midwifery* 2011 Dec; 27(6) 842-7 Available at: www.midwiferyjournal.com/article/S0266-6138(10)00144-0/absract Accessed 23.1.2011

Cheung NF, Chang LP, Mander R, Xu X, Wang X, (2010) Proposed professional education programme for midwives in China: New mothers' and midwives' views. *Nurse Education Today* Available at: www.nurseeducationtoday.com/article/S0260-6917(10)00163-2a abstract Accessed 30.11.2014

Cheung NF, Mander R, Wang X, Fu W, Zhu J (2009) Chinese midwives' views on a midwife-led normal birth unit. *Midwifery* 25(6) :744-755 www.elsevier.com/locate/midw

Cheung NF, (2009) Chinese midwifery: the history and modernity. *Midwifery* 25(3):228-241

Cheung NF, Mander R, Wang X, Fu W, Zhu J (2009) The planning and preparation for a 'homely birthplace' in Hangzhou, China, *Evidence Based Midwifery*, 7(3): 101-106.

Cheung NF, Mander R, Cheng L, Yang XQ, Chen VY (2006b) Caesarean decision-making: negotiation between Chinese women and healthcare professionals. *Evidence Based Midwifery* 4: 24-30.

Cheung NF, Mander R, Cheng L, Chen VY, Yang XQ, Qian HP, Qian JY (2006a) 'Zuoyuezi' after caesarean in China: an interview survey. *International Journal of Nursing Studies* 43(2):193-202.

Cheung NF, Mander R, Cheng L 2005b. The 'doula-midwives' in Shanghai. Evidence Based *Midwifery* 3: 73-79.

Cheung NF, Mander R, Cheng L, Yang XQ, Chen VY (2005a) Informed choice' in the context of caesarean decision-making in China. *Evidence Based Midwifery* 3: 33-8

Department of Health (2012) *Compassion in Practice Nursing, Midwifery and Care Staff Our Vision and Strategy.* Available at: www.england.nhs.uk/wp-content/.../compassion-in-practice.pdf Accessed 6.5.14

Downe S (2011) Identifying progress, gaps and possible ways forward. In Donna S (Ed) *Promoting Normal Birth - Research, Reflections & Guidelines.* Fresh Heart Publishing UK. pp.325-337

Gloucestershire Hospitals (2012) *Nursing and Midwifery Strategy 2013-2015.* Available at: www.gloshospitals.nhs.uk/.../Nursing-Midwifery-Strategy-A4 Accessed 6.5.14

Huang XH 2000. The present and future of caesarean section. *The Journal of the Chinese Applied Obstetrics and Gynaecology* 16(5), 259-261

Mander R, Cheung NF, Wang X, Fu W, Zhu J (2009) Beginning an Action Research Project to Establish a Midwife-Led Normal Birthing Unit in China. *Journal of Clinical Nursing.* 19, (3-4): 517-526 Epub Sep 3, doi:10.1111/j.1365-2702.2009.02849.x Available at: www.ncbi.nlm.nih.gov/pubmed/19732249?dopt=Abstractplus Accessed 30.11.14

World Bank (2013) *HNP Notes* The World Bank.

WHO 2010a Caesarean section without medical indications is associated with an increased risk of adverse short term maternal outcomes: the 2004-2008 WHO global survey on maternal and perinatal health. *BMC Medicine* 8;71, www.biomedcentral.com/1741-7015/8/71

WHO (2010b) Method of delivery and pregnancy outcomes in Asia: the WHO global survey on maternal and perinatal health 2007-08. *The Lancet*, published on-line, January.

Ministry of Health (2012) *China Statistic Yearbook.* Ministry of Health of the Republic of China.

Pan A., Cheung NF (2011) The challenge of promoting normality and midwifery in China. In Donna S (Ed) *Promoting Normal Birth - Research, Reflections & Guidelines.* Fresh Heart Publishing, UK.pp 190-203

Pang Ruyan (2010) [in Chinese] Current status and development of midwifery in China. *Chinese Journal of Nursing Education*, 7; 7, 293-294.

UNFPA (2011) *The state of world's midwifery - delivering health, saving lives.* Available at: www.unfpa.org/sowmy/resources/docs/main_report/en_SOW-MR_Full.pdf Accessed on 30.11.14

UNFPA (2014) *The State of the World's Midwifery 2014. A Universal Pathway: A Woman's Right to Health* New York: United Nations Population Fund

UNICEF (2012) *Maternal and Newborn Health Country Profiles - China.* UNICEF

20 Making it happen in Brazil

Aguiar JM, d'Oliveira AF, Schraiber LB (2013) Institutional violence, medical authority, and power relations in maternity hospitals from the perspective of health workers. *Cadernos de Saude Publica.* 2013 Nov; 29(11): 2287-96. [Article in Portuguese]

Carneiro R (2013) What doctors hardly talk about: trance and ecstasy at the scene of childbirth. Dissident experiences and perceptions of health and welfare in contemporary times. *Ciência e Saúde Coletiva*, 2013; vol.18(8): 2369-2378. [Article in Portuguese] Available from: www.scielo.br/scielo.php?script=sci_arttext&pid=S1413-81232013000800021&lng=en&nrm=iso

D'Oliveira AFPL, Diniz SG, Schraiber LB (2002) Violence against women in health-care institutions: an emerging problem. *The Lancet* 2002; 359: 1681–85

D'Orsi E, Brüggemann OM, Diniz CSG, Aguiar JM, Gusman CR, Torres JA, Angulo-Tuesta A, Rattner D, Domingues RMSM (2014) Social inequalities and women's satisfaction with childbirth care in Brazil: a national hospital-based survey. *Cadernos de Saúde Pública*, 2014; vol.30 (supl.1): S154-S168.

Diniz CSG (2005) Humanization of childbirth care in Brazil: the numerous meanings of a movement. *Ciência e Saúde Coletiva*, 2005; vol.10 (n.3): 627-637. [Article in Portuguese]

Domingues RMSM, Dias MAB, Nakamura-Pereira M TJA, d'Orsi E, Pereira APE, Schilithz AOC; Leal MC. (2014) Process of decision-making regarding the mode of birth in Brazil: from the initial preference of women to the final mode of birth. *Cadernos de Saúde Pública*, 2014; vol.30 (supl.1): S101-S116.

Fundação Perseu Abramo, (2010) *Mulheres Brasileiras e Gênero nos Espaços Público e Privado*. [Article in Portuguese]. Available at: www.apublica.org/wp-content/uploads/2013/03/www.fpa_.org_.br_sites_default_files_pesquisaintegra.pdf

Leal MC, da Gama SGN and da Cunha CB (2005) Racial, socio-demographic, and prenatal and childbirth care inequalities in Brazil, 1999-2001. *Revista de Saúde Pública*, 2005; 39 (1). [Article in Portuguese]

Leal MC, Pereira APE, Domingues RMSM, Theme Filha MM, Dias MAB, Nakamura-Pereira M, Bastos MH, Gama SGN (2014) Obstetric interventions during labour and childbirth in Brazilian low-risk women. *Cadernos de Saude Publica*, 2014; 30 (Supplement): S17-S32.

McCallum C and Reis AP (2006) Re-significando a dor e superando a solidão: experiências do parto entre adolescentes de classes populares atendidas em uma maternidade pública de Salvador, Bahia, Brasil. *Cadernos de Saúde Pública*, 2006; 22(7): 1483-1491. [Article in Portuguese]

Minayo MCS (2006) The inclusion of violence in the health agenda: historical trajectory. *Ciência e Saúde Coletiva*, 2006; 11(2): 375-383. [Article in Portuguese]

Ministry of Health Brazil (1985) [Article in Portuguese] Available at: bvsms.saude.gov.br/bvs/publicacoes/assistencia_integral_saude_mulher.pdf

Ministry of Health Brazil (2011) [Article in Portuguese] Available at: bvsms.saude.gov.br/bvs/folder/rede_cegonha.pdf

Rattner D. (2009) Humanizing childbirth care: pondering on public policies. *Interface (Botucatu)*, *Botucatu*, 2009; v. 13, supl. 1. [Article in Portuguese] Available at: www.scielo.br/scielo.php?pid=S1414-32832009000500027&script=sci_arttext

Schraiber LB, Lucas d'Oliveira AFP, Portella AP Menicucci E (2009) Violência de gênero no campo da Saúde Coletiva: conquistas e desafios. *Ciência e Saúde Coletiva*, 2009; 14(4): 1019-1027. [Article in Portuguese]

Victora C, Aquino EML, Leal MC, Monteiro CA, Barros FC, Szwarcwald CL (2011) Maternal and child health in Brazil: progress and challenges. *The Lancet*, 2011; 377 (9780): 1863 - 1876

Zorzam B, Moreiras Sena L, Franzon AC, Brum K, Rapchan A (2014) *Violência obstétrica - a voz das brasileiras*. [in Portuguese] Available at: www.youtube.com/watch?v=eg0uvonF25M

21 Making it happen in Catalonia, Spain

Department de Salut, Generalitat de Catalunya (2014) *Servei d'Informació i Estudis, Anàlisi de la mortalitat a Catalunya*, 2012. Barcelona

Escuriet R, Pueyo M, Biescas H, Colls C, Espiga I, White J, Espada X, Fusté J, and Ortún V (2014) Obstetric interventions in two groups of hospitals in Catalonia: a cross-sectional study. *BMC Pregnancy and Childbirth* 14:143 .

Ministry of Health, Social Services and Equality (2012) *National Strategy for Sexual and Reproductive Health* Madrid, Spain

22 Italy, where is your beauty?

Ministero della Salute (2011) *Certificato di assistenza al parto (CEDAP). Analisi dell'evento nascita-anno 2010*. Attività editoriali Ministero della Salute. Roma.

McCourt C, Rayment J, Rance S, Sandall J (2014) An ethnographic organisational study of alongside midwifery units: a follow-on study from the Birthplace in England programme. *Health Serv Deliv Res* (7); 2

Reiger K, Dempsey R (2006) Performing birth in a culture of fear: an embodied crisis of late modernity. Health Sociology Review (15); 4, 364-373.

23 A good birth in the Netherlands

De Vries R, Wiegers T, Smulders B, and van Teijlingen E (2009) The Dutch Obstetrical System: Vanguard of the Future in Maternity Care. In Davis-Floyd R, Barclay L, Tritten J, Daviss BA (eds.), *Birth Models That Work*. P 31-54 Berkeley: University of California Press.

De Vries R, Nieuwenhuijze M, Buitendijk S, *et al* (2013) What does it take to have a strong and independent profession of midwifery? Lessons from the Netherlands. *Midwifery*, 29 (10), : 1122-1128.

Spanjer J, de Haan E, Dijk H, Poortman L, Gorter A, de Waal M, de Jong M & Hagens H (1994) *Bevallen en Opstaan. (Birthing and Uprising)* Amsterdam: Uitgeverij Contact.

Van Teijlingen E, Lowis G, McCaffery P & Porter M (Eds.), (2004). *Midwifery and the Medicalization of Childbirth: Comparative Perspectives*. Hauppauge NY: Nova Science Publishers.

24 Open disclosure: a perspective from Ireland

All Ireland Midwifery Conference (2014) *Open Disclosure: Invited views and evaluation,* Joint All Ireland Midwifery Conference, Irish Nurses and Midwives Organisation & Royal College Midwives Northern Ireland, Crown Plaza Hotel, Santry, Dublin. Oct 2014.

Australian Commission on Safety and Quality in Health Care (2008) *Open Disclosure Standard: A National Standard for Open Communication in Public and Private Hospitals, Following an Adverse Event in Health* Care. Sydney: ACSQHC, 2008.

Boothman RC, Blackwell AC, Campbell DA, Commiskey E & Anderson S (2009) A better approach to medical malpractice claims? University of Michigan experience. *J Health Life Sci Law*. 2009'2:125-159

Granger, K (2014) hellomynameis.org.uk

Health Information and Quality Authority (2012) *The National Standards for Safer Better Healthcare*. Dublin, Ireland.

HSE (2014) HSE Open Disclosure Policy: Document Reference Number: QPSD-D-062-1 hse.ie/eng/about/Who/qualityandpatientsafety/nau/Open_Disclosure/opendiscFiles/opendiscpolicyoct13.pdf

Massachusetts Coalition for the Prevention of Medical Errors (2006) *When Things Go Wrong: Responding to Adverse Events. A Consensus Statement of the Harvard Hospitals*. Burlington: Massachusetts Coalition for the Prevention of Medical Errors, 2006.

Murphy M (2013) WHO Patients for Patient Safety Programme 2013 cited in National Patient Safety Agency. (2009a). *Being Open; Saying Sorry When Things Go Wrong*. London: NHS: National Patient Safety Agency 2009.

National Patient Safety Agency (2009b) *Being Open; Saying Sorry When Things Go Wrong*. London: NHS: National Patient Safety Agency 2009. P14

Wu A (2000) Medical error: the second victim *BMJ*. 2000;320:726

Wu A Professor of Health & Policy Management,(2009a) John Hopkins School of Public Health communicating with Geoffrey Hurst, Director Mater health Services, South Brisbane 2009

Wu A Professor of Health & Policy Management, (2009b) John Hopkins School of Public Health communication review of Singapore Academic Hospital 2009.

Wu A (2010) MPH. 5th Annual Duke Medicine Patient Safety and Quality Conference. Johns Hopkins Bloomberg School of Public Health. Jan 2010. www.dukepatientsafetycenter.com/pdf/Being%20Open%20with%20Patients%20and%20Families%20about%20Adverse%20Events.pdf

25 They don't know what they don't know

Aronson L (2013) 'Good' Patients and 'Bad' patients - rethinking our definitions. *New England Journal of Medicine* 369 p796-797

Baker S, Choi P, Henshaw C and Tree J (2005) I felt as though I'd been in Jail; Women's experiences of Maternity Care during labour, delivery and the immediate postpartum. *Feminism Psychology* 15:3 p315-242.

Block J (2007) *Pushed: the painful truth about childbirth and modern maternity care*. Da Capo Press, Cambridge, MA

Coulter A, Locock L, Ziebland S and Calbrese J (2014) Collecting data on patient experience is not enough: they must be used to improve care. *BMJ* 348 p15-17.

de Boer J, Lok A, Van't Verlaat E, Duivenvoorden H, Bakker A and Smit B (2011) Work-related critical incidents in hospital-based health care providers and the risk of post-traumatic stress symptoms, anxiety, and depression: a meta-analysis. *Soc Sci Med* 73:2 p 316-326.

Enkin M (2008) The Seven Stages of Ignorance. *Birth* 35:3, p169-170

Enkin M, Kierse M, Neilson J, Crowther C, Duley L, Hodnett E (2000) *Guide to Effective Care in Pregnancy and Childbirth* (3rd edition). OUP Oxford;

Francis R (2013). *Report of the Mid Staffordshire NHS Foundation Trust public inquiry*. London: The Stationery Office.

Greenhalgh T (2012) Why do we always end up here? Evidence-based medicine's conceptual cul-de-sacs and some off-road alternative routes. *Journal of Primary Health Care* 4:2, p 92-97

Haynes RB, Devereaux PJ and Guyatt GH (2002) EBM 7. March/April p36-38

Health and Social Information Centre (2013) *Hospital Episode Statistics: NHS statistics 2012-2013* Health and Social Information Centre London. Available at: www.hscic.gov.uk/catalogue/PUB12744/nhs-mate-eng-2012-13-summ-re-po-rep.pdf

Higham J (2006) Current themes in the teaching of obstetrics and gynaecology in the United Kingdom *Medical Teacher* Vol. 28: 6, p495–496

Kitzinger S (2005) The Politics of birth. Elsevier London

Lewis P (2013) A house of cards: the futility of a service that fails to listen. *British Journal of Midwifery* 21:3 p158

Lokugamage A (2011) *Heart in the Womb* Docamali Press, London

Lowe N (2014) Dignity in Childbirth *Journal of Obstetric, Gynaecologic and Neonatal Nursing* 43:2 p137-138

Lumsden MA and Symonds IM (2010) New Undergraduate Curricula in the UK and Australia. Best Practice & Research *Clinical Obsterics and Gynaecology* 24 p795-806

Newdick C and Banbury C (2013) Culture, compassion and clinical neglect: probity in the NHS after Mid Staffordshire. *Journal Med Ethics*. Published Online First: 23 May 2013. doi:10.1136/medethics-2012-101048

Patel N and Rajasingam D (2013) User Engagement in the delivery and design of maternity services. Best Practice and Research *Clinical Obsterics and Gynaecology* 27 p597-608.

Prusova K, Tyler A, Churcher L and Lokumage A (2014) Royal Obstetricians Guidelines: How evidence-based are they? *Journal of Obstetrics and Gynecology* June 12 DOI:10.3109/01443615.2014.920794

Regan L (2014) International Women's Day 2014 vimeo.com/92744531

Royal College of Obstetrics and Gynaecology (2009) *National Undergraduate Curriculum in Obstetrics and Gynaecology: report of a working party*. RCOG press London.

Sackett DL, Rosenberg WC, Gray JAM (1986) Evidence based medicine: what it is and what it isn't. *BMJ*. 312:p71–72.

Sandall J, Soltani H, Gates S, Shennan A, Devane D (2013) Midwife-led continuity models versus other models of care for childbearing women (Review). *Cochrane Database of Systematic Reviews*, Issue 8. Art. No.: CD004667. DOI: 10.1002/14651858.CD004667.pub3.

Stone N (2012) Making Physiological Birth Possible: Birth at a freestanding birth centre in Berlin Midwifery 28 p568-575

Symon A (2006) *Risk and choice: Knowledge and Control. Risk and Choice in Maternity Care*. Elsevier London

Tracey S, Hartz D, Tracy M, Allen J, Forti A, Hall B, White J, Lainchbury A, Stapleton H, Beckmann M, Bisits A, Homer C, Foureur M, Welsh A and Kildea S (2013) *The Lancet*. Vol 382, p1723-1732.

Wise J (2013) Litigation in maternity care is rising, says National Audit Office. *BMJ* 347 f6737 www.bmj.com/content/347/bmj.f6737

Wright J D, Pawar N, Gonzalez J S, Lewin S N, Burke W M, Simpson L L, Charles A S, D'Alton M E, Herzog T J (2011). Scientific evidence underlying the American College of Obstetricians and Gynecologists' practice bulletins. *Obstetrics & Gynecology*. 118(3):505-12.

26 With-woman, with-student

Antonovsky A (1979) *Health, Stress and Coping*. San Francisco, Jossey-Bass.

Beck U (1992). *Risk society: towards a new modernity*. Sage Publications Ltd.

Department of Health (2010) *Equity and Excellence: Liberating the NHS*. London, UK: HMSO

Department of Health (2010a) *Midwifery 2020: Delivering expectations*. London, UK: HMSO

Department of Health.(2012) *The NHS Constitution for England*. London, UK: HMSO

DH (2012a) *Compassion in Practice; Nursing, Midwifery and Care Staff, Our Vision and Strategy*, London, UK: HMSO

Dreher D (1996) *The Tao of Personal Leadership*, Harper-Collins, New York.

Eriksson M (2007). *Unravelling the Mystery of Salutogenesis*. Tuku: Folkhalsan Research Centre, Health Promotion Research Programme.

Eva KW, Rosenfeld J, Reiter HI, & Norman GR (2004). An admissions OSCE: the multiple mini-interview. *Medical Education*, 38: 314–326.

Giddens A (1990). *The consequences of modernity*. Cambridge: Polity in association with Blackwell.

Kim S, Phillips WR, Pinsky L, Brock D, Phillips K, Keary,J (2006) A conceptual framework for developing teaching cases: a review of the literature across the disciplines. *Medical Education*: 40: 867 – 876.

Kings Fund (2011) *Report on leadership and management in the NHS*. London, The Kings Fund

Kirkham M (2010). *The midwife-mother relationship* (2nd Ed). Basingstoke: Palgrave-Mcmillan.

Lindstrom B & Eriksson M (2006) Contextualizing salutogenesis and Antonovsky in public health development *Health Promotion International*. 21 (3) pp. 238-244

Lindstrom B & Eriksson M (2010) *The hitchikker's guide to salutogenesis: salutogenic pathways to health promotion*. Helsinki Folkhalsan research center. Health promotion research.

MacKenzie Bryers H & van Teijlingen E (2010). Risk, theory, social and medical models: a critical analysis of the concept of risk in maternity care. *Midwifery*, 26,

488-496.

Mezirow J (1991) Transformative Dimensions of Adult Learning. San Francisco, Jossey-Bass

NMC (2012) *Midwives Rules and Standards*. London NMC

NMC (2011) *The MINT Project*. London, NMC

NMC (2009) *Standards for pre-registration midwifery education*. London, NMC

NMC (2008) *The Code. Standards of conduct, performance and ethics for nurses and midwives*. London, NMC

Rogoff B (1999) Cognitive development through social interaction: Vygotsky and Piaget. In P. Murphy (Ed), *Learners, Learning and Assessment*. London: Open University Press

Salvatori P (2001) Reliability and validity of admissions tools used to select students for the health professions. *Adv Health Sci Educ*, 6:159–75.

Trinh K & Edge W (2012) *Manual for interviewers*. Undergraduate Medical Program Michael G. DeGroote School of Medicine. Ontario: McMaster University.

Williams B (2005) Case Based Learning – a review of the literature: is there scope for this educational paradigm in prehospital education? *Emergency Medicine Journal*, Vol. 22, pp577-581

27 Care and compassion count

Commissioning Board Chief Nursing Officer and Department of Health Chief Nurse Adviser (2012) *Compassion in Practice*. London: DH, NHS Commissioning Board

Department of Health (2013) *NHS Constitution*. London: DH

Hall J (2013) Developing a culture of compassionate care – the midwife's voice? *Midwifery* 29 (2013) 269-271

Hughes AJ, Fraser DM (2010) There are guiding hands and there are controlling hands. Student midwives experience of mentorship in the UK. *Midwifery* 27 477-483

National Perinatal Epidemiology Unit (2010) Delivered with Care: A National survey of Women's Experiences of Maternity Care 2010. Oxford: NEU

Nursing and Midwifery Council (2008) *Standards for Pre-registration Midwifery Education*. London: NMC

Peate I (2012) Kindness, Caring and Compassion. *Australian Nursing Journal* 19 (7) 16

Youngson R (2012) *Time to Care: How to Love Your Patients and Your Job*. Raglan: Rebelheart

29 Moving to positive childbirth

Gjerdingen DK, Froberg DG, Fontaine P (1991) The effects of social support on women's health during pregnancy, labor and delivery, and the postpartum period. *Family Medicine* Jul;23(5):370-5. Available at: www.ncbi.nlm.nih.gov/pubmed/1884933 Accessed on 30.11.14

30 Walking in another's shoes

Nutshell Communications (2014) Available at: www.nutshellcomms.co.uk/ Accessed on: 2.11.14

31 Compassion in the social era

@6CsLive (2014) Empathy so critical Cleveland clinic films excellent youtube.com/watch?v=cDDWvj… Great resource shared on #6CsLive! webinar - TY @KathEvans2 [Twitter] 24 July 2014 Available at twitter.com/6CsLive/status/492302908999081985 Accessed on 16.9.14

Bennett VJ (2014) Join this webinar next week bit.ly/1tHex4Q for #6CsLive week of action on Compassion in Practice pic.twitter.com/zLrEBX-ECHF [Twitter] 16 July 2014 Available at: twitter.com/VivJBennett/status/489334303361613824/photo/1 Accessed on 16.9.14

Byrom S, Byrom A (2013) Social media: Connecting midwives globally MIDIRS *Midwifery Digest* June, Vol 24, No 2

Caremakers (2014) Great piece on #6Cs and #caremakers in the August @theRCN bulletin. Read page 12 Care & Compassion. Download a copy ow.ly/zUz9o [Twitter] 4 August 2014 Available at twitter.com/CaremakersUK/status/496216284707979264 Accessed on 16.9.14

Calvert H (2014) @WeMidwives are community MWs given enough time to show #compassion? 5 min appt, BP, check heart, tick box, out the door #wemidwives [Twitter] 9 September 2014 Available at: twitter.com/HeartMummy/status/509418771094994944 Accessed on 16.9.14

Foord DG (2014) Compassion in Practice: The story so far - @6CsLive webinar 4pm 21 July 6cs.england.nhs.uk/pg/cv_blog/con… #6CsLive #6Cs [Twitter] 10 July 2014 Available at: twitter.com/DGFoord/status/487191849019273216 Accessed 16.9.14

Granger K (2014) Hello my name is [Online] Available at hellomynameis.org.uk/ Accessed on 16.9.14

Haines S (2013) WeNurses Community Blog Compassion in care, student experience 'scared to care' [Online] Available at: wenurses.co.uk/Community-Blog/?p=270 Accessed on 16 .9.14

Marston L (2013) She's off again Compassion: too scared to care [Online] Available from shesoffagaindiaryofastudentnurse.blogspot.co.uk/ Accessed on 16.9.14

Pew Research Internet Project (2014) Social Networking Fact Sheet [Online] Available at: www.pewinternet.org/fact-sheets/social-networking-fact-sheet/ Accessed on 16.9.14

Price A, Price B (2009) Role modelling practice with students on clinical placements *Nursing Standard*, 24(11):51-56

Queen Victoria Hospital (2014) Our patient experience annual report for 2013/14 has been published on our website. ow.ly/3o4xJ4 #6Cs [Twitter] 11 August 2014 Available at twitter.com/qvh/status/498756100251222016 Accessed on 16.9.14

Symplur (2014) The Healthcare Hashtag project #HelloMyNameIs [Online] Available at: www.symplur.com/healthcare Accessed on 16.9.14 hashtags/hellomynameis/analytics/?hashtag=hellomynameis&fdate=09%2F01%2F2013&shour=00&smin=00&tdate=09%2F17%2F2014&thour=00&tmin=00

Vincent E (2014) Homelessness care pathways via @TheQNI #compassion #6Cs

#WeNurses qni.org.uk/docs/Homeless_... [Twitter] 4 August 2014 Available at: twitter.com/emma_rehab/status/496183833134649344 Accessed on 16.9.14

WeMidwives (2014) *Compassionate care: Is it happening?* [Online] Available at: www.wenurses.com/MyNurChat/archive/archivewemidwives09092014.php Accessed 16.9.14

@WeMidwives (2014) Did you see all your bios in a wordcloud shared last night? Thanks for all the tweeting support :) [Twitter] 9 September 2014 (Accessed 16 September 2014) Available from twitter.com/WeMidwives/status/509281390840795136/photo/1

@WeMidwives (2014) @WestburyBecky @HeartMummy time constraints are damaging, but even with 5 mins can try to engage with smile-& lobby for change! [Twitter] 9 September 2014 Available at: twitter.com/WeMidwives/status/509427679058460673 Accessed on 16.9.14)

WeNurses (2013) Can nurses learn compassion? [Online] Available at: www.wenurses.com/MyNurChat/archive/archivewenurses29082013.php Accessed on 16.9.14

Westbury B (2014) @HeartMummy @WeMidwives Totally agree, clinics often run behind as appts not long enough2provide holistic care not just physical #wemidwives [Twitter] 9 September 2014 Available at: twitter.com/MidwifeBec/status/509426939296505856 Accessed on 16.9.14

Westbury B (2014) @WeMidwives @HeartMummy agreed, can still make a difference no matter how short the time spent [Twitter] 9 September 2014 Available at: twitter.com/MidwifeBec/status/509428119267475458 Accessed on: 16.9.14

Yorkshire Evening Post (2014) *A Leeds doctor's simple message which became a global campaign* [Online] Available at: www.yorkshireeveningpost.co.uk/news/latest-news/top-stories/a-leeds-doctor-s-simple-message-which-became-a-global-campaign-1-6692067 Accessed on: 16.9.14

32 Kindness is a cost-effective solution

National Institute for Health and Clinical Excellence (2011) *Costing Report attached to Caesarean Section* (Partial Update of NICE Clinical Guideline 13) www.nice.org.uk/nicemedia/live/13620/57173/57173.pdf Viewed 18th June 2014.

Waitemata District Health Board (2002) Report into the Operating Theatre Fire Accident, Waitakere Hospital, 17th August 2002. *Medsafe*, New Zealand/

Kachalia A, Kaufman SR, Boothman R, Anderson S, Welch K, Saint S, *et al* (2010) Liability claims and costs before and after implementation of a medical error disclosure program. *Annals of Internal Medicine.* 153(4):213-21.

The Mackinnon Partnership (2009) *Identifying the movement of the workforce around the health sector.* www.skillsforhealth.org.uk/component/docman/doc_download/349-turnover-wastage-report.html Viewed 18th June 2014.

Barsade SG, O'Neill OA. (2014) What's Love Got to Do with It? A Longitudinal Study of the Culture of Companionate Love and Employee and Client Outcomes in a Long-term Care Setting. *Administrative Science Quarterly.*

Barsade S ONO. Employees who feel love perform better. *Harvard Business*

Review; 2014. blogs.hbr.org/2014/01/employees-who-feel-love-perform-better Viewed 18th June 2014.

Egbert LD, Battit GE, Welch CE, Bartlett MK. Reduction of Postoperative Pain by Encouragement and Instruction of Patients. A Study of Doctor-Patient Rapport. *The New England Journal of Medicine*. 1964;270:825-7.

Redelmeier DA, Molin JP, Tibshirani RJ. A randomised trial of compassionate care for the homeless in an emergency department. *Lancet*. 1995;345(8958):1131-4.

Stewart M, Brown JB, Donner A, McWhinney IR, Oates J, Weston WW, et al. The impact of patient-centered care on outcomes. *J Fam Pract*. 2000;49(9):796-804.

Bertakis KD, Azari R Patient-centered care is associated with decreased health care utilization. *J Am Board Fam Med*. 2011;24(3):229-39.

Del Canale S, Louis DZ, Maio V, Wang X, Rossi G, Hojat M, *et al*. The relationship between physician empathy and disease complications: an empirical study of primary care physicians and their diabetic patients in Parma, Italy. *Academic Medicine: Journal of the Association of American Medical Colleges*. 2012;87(9):1243-9.

Epilogue: Turning the silence into a roar

Leunig M (2007) *Love and Fear. A Common Prayer*. Available at: spiritedwritings.blogspot.co.uk/2007/10/love-and-fear-michael-leunig.html. Accessed 4th December 2014

Index

#6Cs 203
#hellomynameis 158, 202–3
#realEBM 163
@WeMidwives 199, 205–6
@WeNurses 199, 201

6Cs (Care, Compassion, Competence, Communication, Courage and Commitment) 35, 171, 177, 203
6Cs Live! Campaign 203

Acceptance and Commitment Training (ACT) 26
Active Hope 109
actor midwives 181–8, 210–11
adverse events (when things go wrong)
    and open disclosure 157–61, 212–14
    still-births 38–43, 94, 107
    and students 184
agency staff 24–5
All That Matters Project 194
'allowed'/ 'not allowed' 119, 125, 192
anaesthetists 67–75, 215–16
Anderson, Tricia 148–9
apology, importance of 160, 213, 214
Argentina 134
art, midwifery as 94, 95–6, 103, 145
autonomy
    maternal 123, 165
    professional 105, 107, 109–10, 114

bank staff 24–5
beauty, need for 150–1
behaviours that accompany compassion 21–4
bereavement care 38–43
Big Day Out 210
biobehavioural aspects of birth 163–4
bioethics 28
birth centres see also home-like settings
    in Brazil 138, 139
    in Italy 149–50
    midwives working to save 58–9, 60
birth environment
    beds in hospital settings 103
    in Catalonia 141, 143
    environments of trust 101–3

home-like settings 89, 102, 103, 138, 141, 149–50
    light levels 89, 102, 141
    privacy 80, 83
birth pools 138, 141
Birth Wars, The (McCall) 63
Birthrights 123
Brazil 34–5, 132–9
breastfeeding 49, 87
bringing the best out of everyone 16–20
'bubbles' model of compassion 22–3
bureaucracy 17–18
burn-out (carer), avoiding 16–19, 34–5, 96, 111–15, 214
Burundi 82

6Cs (Care, Compassion, Competence, Communication, Courage and Commitment) 35, 171, 177, 203
caesarean sections
    anaesthetist's perspective 67–8, 72
    in Brazil 134–5, 136, 138–9
    in Italy 147
    mother-requested 30
    in New Zealand 210, 212, 215–18
'calm and connect' response (vs 'fight or flight') 90
Capacitar workshops 109
'care', definitions of 26, 219
care plans, need for flexibility 124
caring for the carers
    avoiding burn-out 16–19, 34–5, 96, 111–15, 214
    compassion for all around 34
    kindness/ support to colleagues 16–19, 108–9
    peer support 159–60, 202
    recognition of emotional impact 19, 25, 111–12, 158–9, 213
    self-care 36, 96, 108–10, 111–15
    self-compassion 35
    staff time-out/ debriefing 25
    support networks for maternity care workers 108–9
    via social media 202
    work-life balance 112–13, 114
'caritas' 12, 95

case-based learning (CBL) 172–6
caseload models 107, 163
Catalonia 140–6
'catching' compassion 67–76, 169–70
categorisation of clients 105–6
Charter for Respectful Maternity Care (White Ribbon Alliance) 28
Check and Challenge process 178–9
China 127–31
choice
    choice of care/ place of care (lack of) 34
    and evidence-based medicine 163
    informed choice 120, 122–6, 142, 193
    law and the choice agenda 122–3
    and risk awareness vs risk aversion 165
clinical guidelines 119–26, 141, 162–3
cognitive behavioural therapy 26
collaborative working see teamworking
communication
    in the 'bubbles' model of compassion 22–3
    choice of language/ words 26, 50–1, 119, 189, 198–9
    facial expressions and body language 92
    importance of 53–6
    and informed choice 123
    and mutual professional support 109
    open disclosure 157–61, 212–14
    skills of 72–3
'compassion', definitions of 21–4, 57–8, 220
Compassion in Practice (DoH) 171
compassion surveys 21
Compassionate Mind, The (Golbert, 2009) 35
Compassionate Mind Training (CMT) 26
confidentiality 80, 83
consent 35, 80, 83, 123
continuity of care 29–30, 33, 107
control, sense of (women's) 28, 72–3, 124
cost-effectiveness of kindness 208–18
courage through compassion 57–61
criminalization of women 134–5
curriculum design (midwife education) 169–76

dads 48–52
dehumanization of birth 119, 133–5 see also dignity; human rights
dementia services, learning from 197–9
detachment vs dissociation 108
difficult patients 24–5, 30, 54, 64, 123, 125–6
dignity, human 27–30, 125, 197
discrimination 80, 83, 134
disempowerment of women 56, 59, 189–95, 197
disrespect and abuse of women 10, 79–85, 134, 165
doctors (obstetricians) 62–6, 208–18
doulas 44–7, 53–6
drama, using 181–8, 210–11

early separation of newborn from mother 143
economic drivers of medicine 165–6, 208–18
efficiency 15–16, 165
embodied knowledge, valuing 109
emotional impact of working in healthcare 19, 25, 111–12, 158–9, 213
empathy 16, 23, 36, 53–5, 57, 67–75, 185, 220
end of life care 28, 94, 196
epidural anaesthesia 28–9, 55, 67, 70–1, 73–4, 89
epigenetics 219–20
episiotomies 55, 134, 136, 148
European Convention on Human Rights 29
Every Woman, Every Child, Every Newborn Action Plan (2014) 82
evidence-based medicine 17, 121–2, 162–3
eye contact 35

Facebook 201 see also social media
facial expressions and body language 92
faith and spirituality 21–2, 94–7
fathers 48–52
fear
    as general driving principle 9–10, 36–7, 98–104
    maternity care providers' fear 98–104, 201–2

and oxytocin 88
and phrases used by professionals 198
tips for dealing with 101
women's fear of childbirth 10, 190–1
Fear becomes Fact cycle 190–2
financial harassment 80, 83
forceps deliveries 55, 63, 134
forum theatre 181–8
Francis Report (Mid Staffordshire NHS Foundation Trust Inquiry) 9, 21, 33–4, 220
freebirth 99
fundal pressure 134

Geréb, Ágnes 45
Good Medical Practice Code (GMC) 125
Granger, Dr Kate 157–61, 202–3
gratitude 71–2
Greenhalgh, Trisha 163
guidelines (clinical) 119–26, 141, 162–3

hand-holding 35
#hellomynameis campaign 158, 202–3
high BMI women 29, 123
'high risk' women 29
history of midwifery 95
holistic principles 94–7, 197
home births 44–7, 49, 59, 102, 137, 153–4
home-like settings 89, 102, 103, 138, 141, 149–50
honesty 40–2, 213
hormones 31–2, 86–93
human dignity principles 27–30, 35, 197
human rights 27–30, 79–85, 164–5
humanization of care 133, 135–6
humour and laughter 69
Hungary 44–7

ICM Gap Analysis 129–30
immobility in labour 103
independent midwives 34, 108–9, 208
individualization of care 122, 124
informed choice 120, 122–6, 142, 193
informed compliance 123
institutional violence 133–5
introducing yourself 70, 72 see also

#hellomynameis
Ireland 157–61
Italy 147–51

job satisfaction 59, 71, 103, 110, 113–14, 128, 143–5
judgemental attitudes, not having 54
judgmental attitudes, not having 40, 64, 159, 191, 215–16

Kenya 81, 84
Kindness Behaviour Training (KBT) 26
Kristeller manoeuvre 134

learning to be caring 67–76, 169–70
light levels 89, 102, 141
listening 24, 53–4, 72, 105, 109
lithotomy position 134
litigation culture 10, 158, 197, 213
Local Supervising Authority Midwifery Officer (LSAMO) 59
long-term consequences of over-medicalized birth 163–4
love letter for midwives 186–7
loving attention 45–6

management of healthcare workers 18–19, 34, 59, 141, 178, 208–18
Maternal Health Vision for Action (USAID 2014) 82
maternal rights charter 83
Maternity Forum (New Zealand) 211
meditation 108
mentoring (midwifery) 33, 58, 177–9
Mexico 134
Mid Staffordshire NHS Foundation Trust Inquiry (Francis Report) 9, 21, 33–4, 220
Midwives Rules and Standards 124
Millennium Development Goals 81, 127
mindfulness 26, 35–6, 108
misogyny 62–4
mobility in labour 103
modesty (vs dignity) 28
mothering the mother 53–6
Multi Mini Interview (MMI) days 170–1
mutual professional support 10, 111–15, 159–60, 186, 202

national maternity agenda 60, 82, 107–8
natural compassion 25, 67, 169–70
Nepal 83
Netherlands 152–6
NICE guidelines 60, 107–8
Nigeria 79, 81, 83–4
Nightingale, Florence 25, 101
NMC Code 124
non-judgemental attitudes 40
non-judgmental attitudes 54, 64, 159, 191, 215–16
nonviolent communication 109
Normal, Better and Positive Birth 35

obese women 29, 123
obstetric violence 133–5, 136
obstetricians 162–7, 208–18
open disclosure 157–61, 212–14
organizational issues 18–19, 96, 106
overdue babies 27
over-medicalization 9–10, 27, 33
oxytocin 86–93, 102–3

partnership working (women and caregivers) 15–20, 48–52, 100–1, 125–6, 198–9
part-time working 106–7
patriarchy 63–5, 125
Patterson, Jenny 109
peer support
    midwives' 159–60, 202
    women-women support 189–95
personalized care 29–30, 106
person-centred practices 48–9
Peru 81–2
physical abuse 80
policies (vs guidelines) 120
policy-led approaches 140–6, 153, 158
Positive Birth Movement (PBM) 189–95
positive deviants 220–1
Post-2015 Development Agenda (ECOSOC 2014) 82
posterior presentations 103
postnatal care 33
praise, of colleagues' achievements 108, 186–7
privacy 80, 83
professional obligations (outside the NHS Trust) 124–5

professional organizations 124, 159–60
professional resilience 111–15, 164
Progress Theatre 181–8
protocols (vs guidelines) 120
public health policies 140–6

qualities of maternity care workers 16–17

rape 31
#realEBM 163
'recommendation,' in guidelines 119–20
recruitment, midwifery 168–76
reflective practice 108–9, 112–13, 203–5
relationships, centrality of 15–20, 96, 100, 106–8, 166, 209–12
resilience, professional 111–15, 164
Resilient Repertoire 113–15
Respectful Maternity Care Charter: The Universal Rights of Childbearing Women (WRA 2011) 83, 84
respectful watching vs intervention 31–2
rights-based approaches 27–30, 79–85
risk-management culture 29–30, 99–100, 122–4, 132–5, 164–5, 197
role modelling 57–8, 108, 169, 177, 203–5

salutogenic approach 169–76
Schwartz rounds 25
self-awareness 26, 96, 108–9, 112–13, 114
self-care 36, 96, 108–10, 111–15
self-compassion 35
self-reliance 154
sexual abuse survivors 185
shared decision making (SDM) processes 119
shortages of midwives 34
skin-to-skin 143
social media 36, 163, 192–3, 199, 201–7
social movements
    in Brazil 136–7
    Positive Birth Movement (PBM) 189–95
South Africa 81
Spain 140–6
spirituality 21–2, 94–7
St George's hospital, Sydney 107

staff surveys 21
staff turnover 214
standardization of medicine 165
stereotyping 106
still-births 38–43, 94, 107
Stork Network (Brazil) 136
student midwives
    curriculum design (midwife
        education) 169–76
    supporting students in practice
        177–80
Supervisors of Midwives (SOMs) 59
support networks for maternity care
    workers 108–9
surveys 21

'tall poppies,' being 60
Tanzania 81, 84
target-setting 17, 165–6
teamworking
    bringing the best out of everyone
        16–20
    centrality of relationships 15–20, 96,
        100, 106–8, 166, 209–12
    collaborative working styles 18, 211,
        215
    following an adverse event 159
    kindness to colleagues 19, 70–1,
        108–9, 186–7
    mutual professional support 10,
        111–15, 159–60, 186, 202
    partnerships (women and caregivers)
        15–20, 48–52, 100–1, 125–6, 198–9
    praising colleagues' achievements
        108, 186–7
    and professional resilience 114
    reducing caesarean rates 215–16
tele-midwifery 128
temporary/ bank/ agency staff 24–5
theatre (drama) 181–8, 210–11
therapeutic touch 90, 92
time
    in definitions of compassion 23
    hospital vs home births 102
    in midwifery services 105
    the precious gift of 54

time-out, need for staff 25
training
    building relationships between
        obstetricians and midwives 210–11
    in Catalonia 141–2
    for doctors 162–7
    learning to be caring 67–76, 202–3
    mentoring (midwifery) 33, 58, 177–9
    for midwives 168–76, 177–80
    using forum theatre 181–8
transparency (open disclosure) 157–61,
    212–14
trauma
    healing via positive birth experiences
        31–2, 137
    taking into account previous trauma
        72–3
triage systems 33
trust 16, 32, 100–2, 123, 211
truthfulness, importance of 40–2, 213
Twitter 36, 163, 199, 201–2, 204–5
'two-to-one' support 128, 130

VBAC (vaginal birth after caesarean)
    134–5
Venezuela 134
vicious circles 15
virtuous circles 205–6
visible leadership programme (VLP) 21
vocations 22, 95

walking in another's shoes 184, 192,
    196–200
water births 138 see also birth pools
@WeMidwives 199, 205–6
@WeNurses 199, 201
White Ribbon Alliance (WRA) 28, 83,
    84
Whittington Health 21–6
Whose Shoes? approach 196–200
words and language, importance of 26,
    50–1, 119, 189, 198–9
work-life balance 112–13, 114
writing, as means of self-care 108

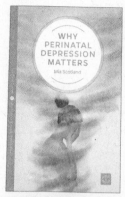
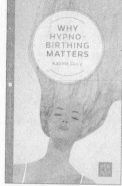
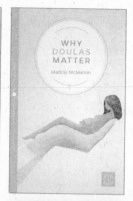
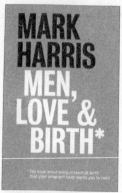
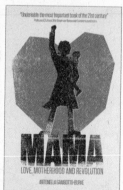
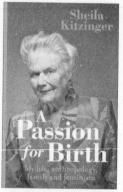
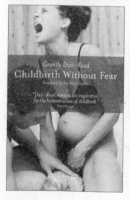
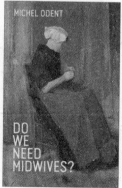
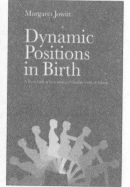